THE COMPASS MODEL IN CRIMINAL AND FORENSIC PSYCHOLOGY

Dr Mark A. Durkin's work developing the COMPASS Model framework is both innovative and needed within Forensic psychological settings. The model emphasises a holistic approach to forensic practice and therefore makes for a more comprehensive approach to understanding and responding to people involved in the criminal justice system. This book introduces the reader to this new framework in detail and is clearly going to be of great use to those seeking to better understand offending populations (students, academics) but also those implementing the model within their forensic practice.

—*Dr Dominic Willmott*, **Reader in Legal and Criminological Psychology, Loughborough University, UK**

Every person has a moral identity consisting of values, norms and principles all of which determine how we think about right and wrong, good and bad etc. However, there are people, trapped in a vicious circle of negative experiences, who are unable to choose and to break loose without help. This book delivers a trustworthy combination of theory and practice as it is based on Dr Durkin's own lived experiences. Through its novel combination of compassion and positive psychology the COMPASS Model will be an excellent practitioner's guide for how to navigate people who wish to make a moral transition in life. With a gentle but instructive voice the author tells the reader how to 'tear down walls' and how to 'build bridges'. This book is an urgent call for unity and understanding in a divided and somewhat incomprehensible world.

—*Dr Mats Niklasson*, **University of Bolton, UK and Vestibularis Clinic, Sweden**

The criminal justice system is a highly complex environment for professionals, the public, and the offender to navigate. Many years of attempted punishment, shaming, reintegration and rehabilitation have created a landscape in which everybody can get lost. Moving forward into new and less damaging futures is fraught with the possibility of losing our way and subsequent failure. By creating this COMPASS model, Durkin builds upon his previous work and brings a fresh perspective to addressing and reducing future offending. The integration of compassion, and the simple but effective visual model, helps describe the journey onwards and upwards. This allows all who travel this route, offenders in particular, to build upon strength and hope, and not wallow in despair and failure. An excellent read!

—*Dr Barrie Green*, RMN, PhD, MA, BA(Hons) (Forensic), PGCert(Law),
DipMDO Forensic Nursing Consultant &
Visiting Research Fellow, University of Bolton

COMPASS is a thought-provoking book that thoroughly unpacks the complex journey of moving away from criminal behaviour. The author combines academic rigor with accessible writing, making it a valuable resource for both students and professionals in Forensic Psychology. The book offers a practical and holistic perspective to desistence and recovery. Engaging, well-structured, and deeply informative, this text is an essential contribution to criminological and psychological literature.

—*Dr Dara Mojtahedi*, PhD, FHEA, C.Psychol Reader
in Forensic Psychology

This book is a very refreshing and eye-opening piece of work! Mark highlights the often-overlooked realities of life's challenges for those with an offending history, and the transformative power of a compassion-focused perspective. Providing examples of personal narratives and offering an insightful analysis, the author describes how their new model can offers a hopeful vision for rehabilitation and reintegration. This book is essential reading for anyone seeking to understand the complexities of the rehabilitation process and the profound impact of compassion and understanding in fostering genuine change.

—*Dr Samantha Marie Walkden* BSc (Hons) MSc PhD CPsychol SFHEA
PGCHE Co-Programme Director MSc Forensic
Psychology, Senior Lecturer in Forensic Psychology

This book is remarkable, unique and innovative at its core. Mark's work incorporates criminological and positive phycological theory, evidence and indeed his own lived experience of receiving criminal justice interventions and desisting from crime. Mark's COMPASS Model constructs a compassionate umbrella, encompassing the leading models within the 'what works' framework. COMPASS provides criminal justice practitioners with an evidence-based tool, integrating and expanding on what is currently known to develop desistance capital, through the recognition of valuing justice involved peoples past, their present and their future. In his own words, the model doesn't claim to know 'what works', but rather draws on 'how it works'. There is no doubt that this book will enhance the knowledge of criminal justice practice at a time when we are in desperate need of innovation.

—*Andrew (Andi) Brierley*, Senior Lecturer, Criminology, Investigation & Policing (CIP)

THE COMPASS MODEL IN CRIMINAL AND FORENSIC PSYCHOLOGY

BY

MARK A. DURKIN
Leeds Trinity University, UK

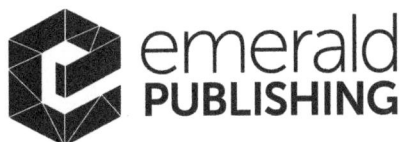

emerald
PUBLISHING

United Kingdom – North America – Japan – India
Malaysia – China

Emerald Publishing Limited
Emerald Publishing, Floor 5, Northspring, 21-23 Wellington Street, Leeds LS1 4DL

First edition 2025

Reprints and permissions service
Contact: www.copyright.com

British Library Cataloguing in Publication Data
A catalogue record for this book is available from the British Library

ISBN: 978-1-83549-557-5 (Print)
ISBN: 978-1-83549-556-8 (Online)
ISBN: 978-1-83549-558-2 (Epub)

Printed and bound by CPI Group (UK) Ltd, Croydon, CR0 4YY

INVESTOR IN PEOPLE

This book is dedicated to my late mother Maureen Durkin,
'love you, see you later'.

CONTENTS

FOREWORD

It is an honour for me to have been asked to write the Foreword for Mark's new book on his exciting Compassionate Positive Applied Strengths-based Solutions (COMPASS) model. I first met Mark in 2012, when I was asked to supervise his undergraduate dissertation in Psychology. We soon developed a close relationship that then led to me supervising his Master's dissertation. He then went on to complete a PhD with me on the topic of compassion. Mark was never someone happy with the status quo. He was always looking to bring in new ideas. He came up with several innovative elements for his doctoral dissertation, including his Compassion Strengths model and his keys for compassion. This book is the culmination of some of these ideas. Mark has brought together the fields of Compassionate Mind Training and the work of Professor Paul Gilbert and himself and combined it with Positive Psychology. COMPASS standing for COM = Compassionate and PASS representing Positive Applied Strengths-based Solutions. He has woven this in with Desistance Capital. This work has not only come from years of scholarship but his own lived experience of having been in the criminal justice system himself. This is what makes this book unique. Mark may well be one of the few people to have entered our penal system and later achieved a BSc an MSc and a PhD in Psychology. Truly, this is a 'redemption narrative'.

Mark starts the book by considering the reasons why people get involved in criminal activity. He covers a range of explanations from biological, psychological and social perspectives. He examines two intervention models in depth. These are the Risk-Need-Responsivity model and the Good Lives Model. The development of his COMPASS model represents a move away from a risk-based approach to working with offenders towards a compassion and strengths-based approach. The notion of desistance capital is also central. Mark draws our attention to human, justice, social and community capital and how each is critical to help people stop re-offending. For Mark, the three key components of the COMPASS model are compassionate understanding of offenders, having a holistic view of desistance and adopting a strengths-based way of working with offenders. In the last chapter, he presents two case studies showing the application of the model.

This book is a welcome addition to the literature on working with offenders. While it seems as if society always wants to punish offenders, the high rates of recidivism show that incarceration in itself is ineffective in the long term. A different set of approaches is needed. The COMPASS model described in this book is an innovative way to engage with offender populations on a more therapeutic basis, rather than from a punitive perspective. The book could have a transformative effect on the criminal justice field. I am delighted to endorse it and its creator, Dr Mark Durkin.

Professor Jerome Carson, September 2024, University of Bolton

ACKNOWLEDGEMENTS

I would like to express my greatest thanks to my friends and family for their unwavering support over the years, especially the ones who were there for me during the worst of times, and indeed while writing this book. To Callum, Megan, Emilia, Eva, Noah, Florence, Nelly, Maggie and Stella for everything you do and all that you are. To my Siany for your love and support. To Professor Jerome Carson for always believing in me. To Andi Brierley for encouraging me to be more open and accepting of my past and to use it as a force for change, thank you brother. To Mahimna Vyas for his extensive review of earlier drafts and to everyone who provided feedback and endorsed the book. To Daniel Ridge for his belief in the idea of the book from our initial meeting and for telling me this book would be a 'game changer'. To everyone at Emerald who has helped in the production of the book and promotion of the ideas within it. Last and by no means least, to anyone who has experience of the justice system, past, present and future, and to everyone who has managed to find their way out of offending, and those who support them along the journey.

1

INTRODUCTION

ABSTRACT

This book presents a novel approach to understanding and addressing offending behaviour through the integration of compassion and positive psychology into a comprehensive model. By drawing on both theoretical frameworks and personal experience, the book offers a unique perspective on criminal justice and desistance. The author, having navigated the complexities of offending and incarceration, provides an authentic voice that bridges lived experience with academic insight. The book introduces the COMpassionate Positive Applied Strengths-based Solutions (COMPASS) model, which combines elements of compassion-focused therapy, positive psychology, capital and desistance theory to create a holistic guide for practitioners and individuals within the criminal justice system.

Keywords: Lived experience; offending behaviour; prisons; compassion; positive psychology

INTRODUCTION

The text is structured into three main sections: the past, the present and the future. It begins with an exploration of offending theories and current models, progresses through the principles of compassion and positive psychology and culminates in a practical application of the COMPASS model with real-life case studies. This integrative approach aims to address the systemic issues of offending and re-offending by focusing on the human potential for change, leveraging both compassion and positive psychology to foster effective desistance. Ultimately, the book aspires to offer a theoretical framework and a practical guide that reflects the lived experiences of those who have been through the criminal justice system. It seeks to inspire and equip practitioners to support meaningful change, emphasising that compassion and positive psychology can significantly enhance the process of desisting from crime and improving outcomes for individuals and communities alike.

MOTIVATION FOR THIS BOOK

The impetus for writing this book stems from a deep-seated desire to contribute positively to the justice system, informed by both my personal experiences and academic insights. Drawing from my own encounters with the criminal justice system, coupled with my educational journey, I aim to present a compassionate, positive strengths-based approach to addressing the systemic issues plaguing justice systems globally. Recent statistics underscore the urgency of reforming how we address offending and re-offending. The Office for National Statistics (ONS) Crime Survey for England and Wales reported approximately 8.8 million offences in March 2024, with similar trends observed in the United States (FBI Crime Data Explorer, 2024). In Australia, there were 347,742 offences with most acts of harm to others (26%), illicit drug offences (15%) and public order offences (11%) (Australian Bureau of Statistics, 2024). Crime affects all societal layers, exacting a heavy psychological and emotional toll on victims and their families. For instance, surviving a loved one's murder involves a complex grief process with lifelong repercussions, while robbery or theft can lead to severe anxiety and altered daily behaviours. Families of offenders often face stigma and shame, compounding the broader impact of criminal behaviour.

I believe that a paradigm shift towards compassion and positive psychology could help mitigate these issues. Just as one act of crime can have far-reaching negative effects, a unified approach grounded in compassion and positive psychology has the potential to foster significant positive change, both in reducing crime and alleviating the suffering it causes.

THE VALUE OF LIVED EXPERIENCE

One of the driving forces behind this book is recognising that many rehabilitation models lack input from those with first-hand experience in the criminal justice system. Those who have lived through the challenges of offending and incarceration offer invaluable insights that can be used to support the desistance of people who offend and improve justice practice (Brierley, 2023; Buck, 2020). Integrating these lived experiences with academic research can provide a comprehensive framework for addressing offending behaviour. This book aims to bridge this gap by drawing on personal experiences and academic research to propose a novel approach to criminal justice that addresses the root causes of offending with compassion and fosters positive meaningful change.

PERSONAL INSPIRATION

The inspiration for this book is deeply rooted in my own experiences with the criminal justice system. Incarcerated from ages 19 to 21 for drug offences, my journey took a transformative turn at 31 when I enroled in an access course to higher education in psychology. Despite having no formal qualifications and facing numerous challenges, I then pursued a bachelor's degree, a master's and a PhD in Psychology. My personal journey from incarceration to academia underscores the potential for change and the impact of compassion, hope, gratitude, strength and support. This book not only aims to offer a practical guide for practitioners working with offenders but also to serve as a source of inspiration for those who may feel trapped by their past. By demonstrating that profound personal transformation is possible, I hope to encourage both people who have offended and practitioners to believe in and work towards positive change.

HOW WE TREAT OFFENDING BEHAVIOUR?

Traditionally, criminal behaviour is met with punitive measures, rooted in longstanding moral and religious notions of good and evil. There are approximately 11 million people held in prisons across the world either on remand or sentenced (Fair & Walmsley, 2024), with the United Nations Office on Drugs and Crime (2024), reporting that incarceration rates are on the rise. Prisons are overcrowded, and nearly a third of offenders are in pre-trial detainment, with 1 in 10 deaths a result of suicide. The United States leads the global incarceration rates, with over 2 million people sent to prison across all states (World Population Review, 2024). The incarceration of offenders comes at a significant social and economic cost. In the United Kingdom, for example, the annual cost of housing a prisoner is approximately £49,000, with re-offending rates contributing to a financial burden exceeding £18 billion annually (PRT, 2021). This underscores the pressing need for effective rehabilitation and reintegration strategies. The Netherlands and various Scandinavian nations have demonstrated the benefits of focusing on normalising prison life to reflect the outside world and treating inmates as people over and above confinement and incarceration (van de Rijt et al., 2023). These countries have significantly reduced recidivism rates by integrating programmes that address the root causes of offending and support reintegration (Boone et al., 2022). The United Kingdom's current approach includes early releases to manage prison overcrowding, yet this also highlights the need for comprehensive support plans for all individuals involved. As rule four of the Nelson Mandela Rules (United Nations, 2015, p. 3) states:

> *The purposes of a sentence of imprisonment or similar measures depriving of a person's liberty are primarily to protect society against crime and to reduce recidivism. Those purposes can be achieved only if the period of imprisonment is used to ensure, so far as possible, the reintegration of such persons into society upon release so that they can lead a law-abiding and self-supporting life.*

Prisons, as institutions, present a paradox. They aim to protect society by isolating offenders, yet this environment can facilitate the formation of criminal networks and escalate offending behaviour. While some prisons offer educational and vocational programmes that aid desistance, their effectiveness varies widely. Alternatives to incarceration, such as community-based supervision, also require robust support systems to be successful. Furthermore, current 'offender rehabilitation' models do not identify or pinpoint where barriers to desistance and problems with re-offending may occur and whether this is at a personal, social, justice or community level. Knowing this could help policymakers and those working with offenders make more informed decisions about interventions to prevent offending behaviour. The COMPASS model presented in this book departs from a predominately risk-based approach to a compassionate and strengths-based approach to the treatment of justice involved people.

The professionals working within the justice system – probation officers, social workers and counsellors, play a critical role in fostering hope and facilitating change. Their interactions with offenders can significantly impact the desistance process, though they too face challenges such as burnout and systemic limitations. Efforts are needed to ensure that desistance support starts at the beginning of a prison sentence and continues all the way through the incarceration period to release and then further in the community. Staff need to be supported along this journey and theirs as well as inmates' perspective considered so that prisons can be designed with everyone's needs in mind and foster a holistic approach to desistance and the prevention of offending.

MOVING FORWARD WITH COMPASSION AND POSITIVE PSYCHOLOGY

Our approach to criminal behaviour should transcend mere punishment and aim to address the underlying causes of offending. Offending behaviour often stems from complex personal histories that are overlooked in traditional punitive approaches. Viewing offending through a compassionate lens allows us to recognise the humanity in every individual and understand the broader context of their actions. Compassion, both from others and towards oneself, has been a transformative force in my own life. It is a critical element often missing from forensic and criminal psychology but is essential for fostering meaningful change. This book aims to advocate for a justice system that is both compassionate and effective, focusing on reducing offending and sup-porting desistance through a compassionate, human-centred approach that moves away from a rigid didactic view of offending to one that considers the interplay of multiple factors involved in offending behaviour.

This book offers a fresh perspective on criminal justice, emphasising the need for a compassionate and holistic approach to dealing with offending behaviour. By prioritising humane treatment and supportive interventions, we can work towards a justice system that not only addresses criminal behaviour but also promotes lasting positive change.

AIMS OF THE BOOK

The primary aim of this book is to introduce and elaborate on a new model for understanding offending behaviour and supporting individuals in their journey towards desistance. Grounded in the author's personal experience with the criminal justice system and informed by contemporary evidence from compassion and positive psychology, the book presents the COMPASS model.

STRUCTURE OF THE BOOK

The book is divided into three main sections across eight chapters:

Past: This section lays the groundwork by exploring theories on why people offend and reviewing current models aimed at reducing offending behaviour.

Chapter 1: Introduction to the book, author background, and a rationale for moving forward with compassion and positive psychology.

Chapter 2: Examination of key theories on offending, including evolutionary perspectives from compassion-focused therapy.

Chapter 3: Review of existing frameworks like Risk Need Responsivity and Good Lives Model, highlighting their strengths and limitations.

Present: This section delves into contemporary theories and practices relevant to the COMPASS model.

Chapter 4: Exploration of Compassion-Focused Therapy (CFT) and its application in understanding and addressing offending behaviour.

Chapter 5: Overview of positive psychology principles and their role in enhancing well-being and life satisfaction.

Chapter 6: Discussion of desistance theory and the concept of desistance capital.

Future: The final section integrates previous theories into the COMPASS model and provides practical examples.

Chapter 7: Introduction to the COMPASS model.

Chapter 8: Case study examples demonstrating the application of the COMPASS model in practice.

INTENDED AUDIENCE AND USE

This book is for practitioners within the criminal justice system and anyone involved in supporting individuals who have offended. It provides an integrative approach combining compassion-based and positive psychology interventions with capital and desistance theory, offering a holistic perspective on offending behaviour. By understanding the complexities of why people offend and the factors that influence their behaviour, readers will be better equipped to support individuals in achieving positive change and leading pro-social lives.

CONCLUSION

This book stands out for two key reasons. First, it integrates compassion and positive psychology into a comprehensive model designed to guide practitioners, individuals who have offended and those working within the criminal justice system. This holistic approach is intended to offer practical, compassionate strategies for fostering desistance and promoting positive change. Second, it is informed by my own lived experience with offending, incarceration and the criminal justice system. Having navigated the complexities of crime, prison life and the associated stress and stigma, I offer a perspective that is both personal and practical. My journey from a troubled past to a successful career in psychology exemplifies the potential for transformation and underscores the impact of compassion and positive psychology. I am living proof that change is not only possible but also profoundly transformative. Moments of compassion, hope and optimism have been pivotal in my own life, enabling me to make critical changes and achieve my current position. Through this book, I blend theory, practice and personal experience in a way that is both engaging and instructive. By doing so, I hope to provide valuable insights and tools for those working with individuals who have offended, demonstrating how compassion and positive psychology can enhance effective practice and support meaningful, lasting change.

REFERENCES

Australian Bureau of Statistics. (2024). *Recorded Crime – Offenders*. https://www.abs.gov.au/statistics/people/crime-and-justice

Boone, M., Pakes, F., & van Wingerden, S. (2022). Explaining the collapse of the prison population in the Netherlands: Testing the theories. *European Journal of Criminology*, *19*(4), 488–505.

Brierley, A. (2023). An introduction to the team and project. In A. Brierley (Ed.), *The good prison officer* (pp. 1–16). Routledge.

Buck, G. (2020). *Peer mentoring in criminal justice*. Routledge.

Fair, H., & Walmsley, R. (2024). *World prison population list*. ICPR.

Federal Bureau of Investigation. (2024). *FBI Crime Data Explorer*. https://cde.ucr.cjis.gov/LATEST/webapp/#/pages/home

Office for National Statistics. (2024). *Crime in England and Wales: Year ending March 2024.* https://www.ons.gov.uk/peoplepopulationandcommunity/crimeandjustice/bulletins/crimeinenglandandwales/yearendingmarch2024

Prison Reform Trust. (2021). *Bromley briefing prison factfile: Winter 2021.* https://www.prisonreformtrust.org.uk

United Nations. (2015). *Standard minimum rules for the treatment of prisoners.* (The Nelson Mandela Rules). https://www.un.org/en/events/mandeladay/mandela_rules.shtml

United Nations Office on Drugs and Crime. (2024). *Global prison population and trends: A focus on rehabilitation.* https://www.unodc.org/documents/data-and-analysis/briefs/Prison_brief_2024.pdf

van de Rijt, J., van Ginneken, E., & Boone, M. (2023). Lost in translation: The principle of normalisation in prison policy in Norway and the Netherlands. *Punishment & Society*, 25(3), 766–783.

World Population Review. (2024). *Incarceration rates by country.* https://worldpopulationreview.com/country-rankings/incarceration-rates-by-country

2

THE BIOPSYCHOSOCIAL REASONS FOR WHY PEOPLE OFFEND

ABSTRACT

This chapter delves into the biopsychosocial reasons behind offending behaviour. It provides an overview of key theories from the biological, psychological and social perspectives in psychology and criminology. The discussion includes different viewpoints on why people offend, focusing on Compassion-Focused Therapy and positive psychology. It explores how these approaches contribute to our understanding of offending behaviour.

Keywords: Biopsychosocial; ACEs; psychology; sociology; biology

THE BIOPSYCHOSOCIAL REASONS FOR WHY PEOPLE OFFEND

There are several key theories to describe and understand the causes of crime and reasons for why people offend that can be broadly categorised into biological, psychological or sociological. Each one will be covered briefly in this chapter.

BIOLOGICAL

Biological theories of criminal behaviour assume that there is an inherent explanation for why someone engages in crime. They draw on genetics, brain mechanisms and psychophysiology theory to explain criminal behaviour. Earlier biological theories proposed that some people were born criminals (Lombroso, 1876), yet more recent developments have shown that a more comprehensive explanation of the reasons people offend is needed.

GENETICS

Research suggests that intelligence, mental health and personality, which are thought to be related to criminal behaviour, are hereditary (Baker et al., 2006). Evidence for the association of genetics and criminal behaviour has grown over the years, with twin studies providing a better understanding of the links between genes and their environments (Glenn & Raine, 2014). Gard et al. (2019) found that although being anti-social was hereditary, it differed between age and behaviour subtypes, with non-shared environmental factors such as Adverse Childhood Experiences (ACEs), parental incarceration and disadvantaged neighbourhoods, showing more variance between genes and anti-social behaviour. Genes are usually activated in different contexts and can influence a person's sensitivity to environmental stressors (Ling et al., 2019). Gene × Environment (G × E) interactions can increase the risk factors associated with offending behaviour. This can help to explain how two people growing up in the same neighbourhood where crime is common may go in different directions, with one engaging in crime and the other not. Their genes make them susceptible to criminal behaviour due to the environment they grow up in and live in. For example, people who have experienced ACEs are more likely to exhibit symptoms of trauma and offending behaviour in later life (Zannas et al., 2015), males being more susceptible to offending and females to symptoms of depression (Wright & Schwartz, 2021).

The Evolutionary Neuroandrogenic (ENA) theory also supports claims for the link between biology and criminal behaviour (Ellis & Hoskin, 2015). Extending Darwin's theory of evolution by natural selection and gene theory, ENA suggests that males display greater competitive/victimising behaviours than females because male's brains develop differently to females. Females are more likely to mate with males who are seen as skilled providers of resources. Competitive/victimising behaviours fall on a continuum of very crude to very sophisticated, with crude behaviours explaining some criminal behaviour. Very crude behaviours require hardly any skills or learning and are classed as street crimes such as assaults, confiscatory or minor drug offences. These acts are considered intentional behaviours that seek to harm or take from others. On the other hand, the very sophisticated crimes require more organisation, complex learning and thought. This side of the continuum includes business ventures where people in management are paid more than the workers, as in all capitalist structures. The competitive nature of human beings has been applied to the compassion-focused understanding of human behaviour and can be considered critical for explaining the biological mechanisms associated with offending and the ability to regulate emotions (Gilbert, 2007).

BRAIN MECHANISMS

Offending behaviour is associated with the pre-frontal cortex (PFC) area of the brain, which is responsible for executive functioning such as attention, emotional regulation, decision-making, moral reasoning and impulse control (Sapolsky, 2004). Impaired functioning in this area of the brain is associated with offending and anti-social behaviour (Meijers et al., 2017). Further support for the link between the PFC and offending behaviour comes from research into transcranial stimulation of the PFC, with results showing an increase in the moral implications of aggressive acts and a decrease in the drive to offend (Choy et al., 2018). It is worth noting here that these issues with the PFC are not always present among all offender groups. For example, white-collar criminals do not display the same deficits as blue-collar criminals (Ling & Raine, 2018). Successful psychopaths also do not have the same reduced volume of brain areas as unsuccessful psychopaths (Yang et al., 2015), suggesting that these areas of the brain differ for types of offenders.

The amygdala is another significant part of the brain that is thought to be responsible for criminal behaviour. This area of the brain is associated with emotional processing especially negative emotions and threat-based facial and auditory expressions in non-offenders and in both violent and non-violent offenders (Zeng et al., 2022). A healthy amygdala is involved with stimulus-reinforcement learning and teaches us about fear to avoid risky situations and recognise cues of distress in others so that we learn not to inflict hurt on them. This deters many from getting involved in criminal behaviour. However, the ability to identify threats or distress in others diminishes because of amygdala maldevelopment and increases the likelihood of offending and anti-social behaviour (Ling & Raine, 2018).

Stress and trauma are key factors that reduce the volume of the amygdala. Post-traumatic stress disorder (PTSD) affects a considerable proportion of inmates, and while the prison environment can influence the symptoms, it is argued that many prisoners already have these symptoms prior to entering the prison system (Facer-Irwin et al., 2022), which are associated with ACEs. Svingen (2023) suggests that exposure to trauma makes the amygdala hypersensitive to perceived threat and someone more prone to aggressive criminal behaviour but is often overlooked as a reason for why people offend. Considering this from the perspective of Compassion-Focused Therapy (CFT), a person would have an increased threat system and respond to environmental stimuli with anxiety, fear or aggression.

The striatum is a further area of the brain that is linked to offender behaviour. It is associated with reward and emotional processing (Glenn & Yang, 2012), and increased activity is related to impulsivity and offending behaviour (Geurts et al., 2016). For example, in relation to heated interactions with others, having the ability to suppress anger and threat-based impulses helps us to control our aggressive reactions. While research tends to focus more on individuals with psychopathic traits, violent offenders with elevated levels of aggression also demonstrate that more activity occurs in the striatum when they are aggravated than in non-offenders (da Cunha-Bang et al., 2017). An imbalanced drive system or a threat/drive system would explain the increase in aggression, impulsive behaviour and the need for reward. It also indicates how working on the soothing system could help regulate emotions and limit aggressive responses during interactions with others.

ADVERSE CHILDHOOD EXPERIENCES (ACES)

The origin of ACEs can be found in a groundbreaking study that explored three types (physical and emotional abuse, neglect and household dysfunction) of specific adversity that occur in the home prior to a person's 18th birthday in relation to outcomes later in their life (Felitti et al., 1998). ACEs can create a sense that the world is a hostile and unsafe place to live. Many resort to maladaptive pathological behaviours to alleviate the emotional/cognitive dissonance and shame that arise from their adverse experiences leading them to a path of offending behaviour (Sajadian et al., 2024). People who experience ACEs are more likely to develop mental health issues and be involved in offending (Turner et al., 2021). Studies with offender groups found that a high number of ACEs were related to criminal behaviour, prompting the need for interventions aimed at helping people desist from offending to focus on past experiences (Reavis et al., 2013) and protective factors such as school attainment, low impulsivity and emotional regulation that could moderate the effects of ACEs on offending behaviour (Craig et al., 2017). Malvaso et al. (2022) suggested 87% of people involved in the criminal justice system experienced at least one ACE, with 12% reporting experiences of sexual abuse and 80.4% parental separation. A more recent meta-analysis found that ACEs associated with abuse were more prevalent among female offenders, and overall neglect was linked to an increase in offending for both genders (Astridge et al., 2023). The authors of this study suggested that although a greater number of ACEs was almost 100% associated with risk factors related to re-offending, each should be considered individually concerning its impact on the person.

INTERACTION OF BIOLOGICAL FACTORS

The Neuro-Moral Theory of anti-social behaviour was first put forward by Raine and Yang (2006). This theory suggests that different areas of the brain other than the PFC, amygdala and striatum overlap to explain offending behaviour. According to this theory, offending behaviour exists on a spectrum, with offences such as proactive aggression (actively seeking out or driven towards aggression as a reward), primary psychopathy at the higher end and secondary psychopathy, drug offences, and reactive aggression at the lower end. Integration of the PFC and the amygdala is connected to moral behaviour, with both participating in the self-regulation of emotions, thoughts and behaviours and are connected to the autonomic nervous system that is responsible for heart rate and breathing. One of the aims of CFT is to regulate the emotional systems by developing a compassionate self and the ability to self-soothe (Gilbert, 2009). Thus, learning to regulate emotions, thoughts and behaviour using the skills of compassion could help control offending behaviour at the biological level.

PSYCHOPHYSIOLOGY

Psychophysiological explanations of offending behaviour refer to two fundamental areas of arousal that can be measured: skin conductance (sweat rate) and heart rate. Both relate to the autonomic nervous system. Heart rate is associated with both the sympathetic and parasympathetic nervous system and skin conductance the sympathetic. A blunted autonomic nervous system is said to be a causal factor in offending behaviour (Choy et al., 2018). Known as the 'Fearlessness Hypothesis', the blunting effect creates a state of discomfort that prevents the person from experiencing the usual physiological responses to risky or stressful situations, so they engage in criminal behaviours to raise their arousal levels (Raine, 2002). Resting heart rate is considered the best predictor of anti-social behaviour, with larger effect sizes observed for psychopathy and violent offenders and smaller for anti-social behaviour and aggression (de Looff et al., 2022). For skin conductance, high levels of proactive aggression are associated with lower fear conditioning in late teens among people who offend but not with reactive aggression (Gao et al., 2015). Therefore, psychophysiological explanations seem to be different, with elevated autonomic responses more prevalent in violent and those driven towards aggressive tendencies.

Addressing these imbalances through emotional regulation interventions may help reduce aggression (Sousa et al., 2022).

Biological theories offer insights into criminal behaviour, but genetic studies have limitations and cannot fully explain human complexity. Genetics should be considered alongside environmental and social factors. For instance, individuals from the same high-crime area may act differently due to unique genetic-environment interactions. Brain abnormalities vary among offenders, suggesting different neurological origins for different crimes. Additionally, violent offenders often show heightened physiological responses. Addressing these imbalances through emotional regulation interventions may help reduce aggression. The correlation between high numbers of ACEs and criminal behaviour highlights the importance of trauma-focused interventions.

PSYCHOLOGICAL

Five major theories cover the psychological theory of crime and offending behaviour: Psychodynamic, cognitive (behavioural), intelligence and personality.

PSYCHODYNAMIC THEORY OF CRIME

Psychodynamic theories propose that criminal behaviour occurs because of early childhood experiences, such as being neglected or lacking any nurturing other to aid in moral development. This theory is based on Freud's ideas of the id, ego and super-ego. The id is the part of the brain that develops from birth and is driven by the desire for primitive needs, such as sex, food and shelter. Freud referred to this as the pleasure principle in which, desires, needs and instant gratification need to be met. Because of this instant need for things, no matter what the cost, the id is explained as the cause of criminal deviance. In relation to the drive system and the acquisition of capital, the purpose of the ego is to seek out the id's desires in the person's environment. The super-ego contains all the persons' moral knowledge of rights and wrongs learned from parents or carers during development. The ego's other purpose is to balance the id's desires and the moral wishes of the super-ego. This helps reduce feelings of shame and guilt while projecting the ideal self into society, also found in those who regulate emotions with compassion and self-soothing exercises (Gilbert, 2009). Shame and humiliation can act as motivators for serious violent crime where the projection of rage onto inanimate objects escalates to people as a way of ridding the violent person of unwanted feelings brought on by loss, trauma and parental neglect (Jump & Gray, 2024). Thus, people do not simply engage in criminal behaviour because they are bored or frustrated by the lack of opportunity in their environment. There is an internal as well as an external cause for offending behaviour.

COGNITIVE (BEHAVIOURAL) THEORY

Cognitive theory considers criminal and pro-social behaviour to be the result of cognitive processes such as moral development and cognitive distortions. Moral development is considered a key cognitive construct in understanding offending behaviour. We all have a moral compass directing us towards what we consider to be good behaviour and away from what is considered bad or unethical behaviour. If we were born alone, we would have no one else to be bad with and only be able to harm ourselves. Therefore, morality is a social cognitive concept driven by our relationships with others and how we behave towards them. According to the literature, it contains moral judgement, empathy, shame and guilt within it. Exclusions from the social group can lead to feelings of shame and a threat to the moral identity of the individual (Gilbert, 2017). Defensiveness can become the action of the person who has offended as a response to alleviate feelings of shame but in a negative way. Based on Kohlberg's (1971, pp. 24–84) theory of cognitive development of moral judgement, external forces such as the avoidance of punishment help establish lower states of moral judgement in the initial stages of development. This helps children learn about accepted social norms, rules, laws and the right way to behave in a safe society. Higher states develop later in life and include the ability to reason with others and create mutual trust and respect as well as reciprocity. An unwritten social contract is developed with a shared under-standing of the social rules to be followed within society.

To perceive another's internal state also includes a cognitive element, which is referred to as perspective-taking in empathy literature (Davis, 1983). Moral judgements are prevalent in people who offend, with lower states responsible for anti-social and offending behaviour (Van Vugt et al., 2011). Emotional states of empathy, shame and guilt underpin moral development and help motivate moral judgements. The ability to understand the impact of the action on another person's feelings and feel something in return is fundamental to moral development and pro-social behaviour and can be developed through compassion-focused practices.

Cognitive distortion is a term that describes offence-supporting attitudes and cognitive processes that are used to justify offending behaviour (Maruna & Mann, 2006). The distinct types of cognitive distortions associated with offending behaviour are minimisation, denial and justification (Ó'Ciardha & Ward, 2013). Some refer to these collectively as a pro-criminal attitude because they are self-serving cognitive distortions that externalise problems (Banse et al., 2013). Such cognitive distortions and the externalisation of problems are linked to Seligman's work on attributional styles, where someone places the blame for failures on external attributions and success on internal attributions. However, research shows that people who create external excuses for negative life events are more likely to maintain their self-esteem, be happier and avoid stress and anxiety (Seligman & Elder, 1986). In fact, Maruna (2004) found similar attribution styles to people with depression among desisting and active offenders, with those actively offending exhibiting signs of learned helplessness and no hope of stopping their offending behaviour. These findings also relate to moral functions of shame and guilt with guilt-based externalisation associated with doing a 'bad thing' and shame-based intern-alised feelings of being a 'bad person' because the offence was committed.

While they can be thought of as simply excuses, Maruna and Mann (2006) argue that cognitive distortions can function as 'windows into the mind' of the offender and reveal more about their criminogenic needs and risk factors. They use the example of someone blaming stress for their offending, as being a way of recognising that the person needs support with regulating their emotional responses to stresses in their life. Practitioners can easily judge through a critical lens and see them as excuses for avoiding taking responsibility for offending behaviour. Moving away from this form of judgemental to a non-judgemental compassionate perspective can be liberating for both offender and practitioner. Probing the excuse together can help explore and address some of the underlying cognitive and other psychological issues associated with offending that lie below the surface that can be used to reduce risks and to explore avenues for change.

From a cognitive perspective, criminal behaviour is preceded by thoughts of offending. Criminal thinking is considered a strong predictor of offending behaviour and is defined as the cognitive process and thoughts that encourage the beginning and maintenance of offending behaviour (Walters, 2006). Andrews et al. (2006) define criminal thinking as the attitudes, beliefs and values that support offending behaviour. These attitudes and thinking styles can be formed in social associations with other offenders and were first referred to in Sutherland's Differential Association Theory (1934, 1937, 1949) who proposed that criminal behaviour was learned and normalised through peers. Those who possess criminal thinking patterns and attitudes towards crime will normalise their offending as being a way of life (Walters, 2006). Criminal thinking styles are associated negatively with pro-social behaviour, and pro-criminal behaviour is more likely to continue when the person denies responsibility for their offence (Martí-Vilar et al., 2019; Maruna & Copes, 2005).

In identifying the thinking patterns associated with offending behaviour, Walters (1995) proposed eight thinking patterns that are present in a criminal lifestyle: mollification (rationalisation and placing blame on external factors), cut-off (rapidly disregarding feelings that prevent from anti-social acts), entitlement (they can take or do whatever they want), power orientation (the need for control over the other people), sentimentality (good deeds to offset depressing feelings about committed crime), super-optimism (confidence of avoiding the negative result of a committed crime), cognitive indolence (lack of developed mental strategies) and discontinuity (lack of determination and consistency in thinking and behaviour). When we look at these thinking styles, they are based on self-serving, irrational and impulsive needs for instant gratification and demonstrate an active threat/drive system.

RATIONALE CHOICE THEORY

Rational choice theory considers offending behaviour as the thinking that develops when deciding to commit a crime. The person will go through a four-choice process. The first is whether to commit a crime or not; the second is who the target should be; third, how often to offend; and fourth, whether they want to persist with or desist from crime (Cornish & Clarke, 1987). Evidence for this theory has been found with juvenile offenders when making the choice to engage in either theft or fighting. Zhao et al. (2021) found that when making the decision, a cost-benefit process occurs where they weigh up the benefits of the offence against the risks and consequences of being caught.

PERSONALITY

Theories such as the Five Factor Model (FFM) and Psychopathy focus on personality traits associated with offending behaviour. The FFM identifies low conscientiousness and high neuroticism as risk factors for offending (Miller & Lynam, 2003). Psychopathy, characterised by traits such as callousness, manipulativeness and egocentricity, correlates with criminal behaviour (Hare, 2003).

Understanding personality traits provides insight into the likelihood of offending and the effectiveness of therapeutic interventions. In a meta-analysis of the literature, Tharshini et al. (2021) found that individual personality traits of psychopathy, low self-control and difficult temperament all contributed to offending behaviour but were predicated on things such as ACEs, environmental factors and poor attachment and emotional regulating systems.

Critics of personality theories argue that because they predict that people with these traits will become offenders and the only way to address this is through incarceration, they fail to consider that personality is malleable or that other social factors may contribute to offending behaviour (Jolliffe & Farrington, 2024). We now know that personality can change over a person's lifetime and that certain interventions can help. Interventions that can aid in personality changes are based on Cognitive Behavioural Therapy (CBT) and humanistic approaches or a blend of both (Roberts et al., 2017). Developing compassion may help people become more agreeable, which is a promotive factor that predicts a lower chance of offending (Jolliffe & Farrington, 2024) through emotional regulation, understanding attachment and the impact of ACEs and shame on anti-social behaviour (Garbutt et al., 2023).

ATTACHMENT THEORY

John Bowlby (1958) developed the theory of attachment to explain the maternal bond between mother/caregiver and child and the developmental impact this has on the child when separated. According to Bowlby, carers represented a 'secure base' to which the children could explore the world around them safely, knowing they could return for comfort when distressed. Without this, they would struggle to meet their needs, which would inhibit their normal development. Bowlby (1988) proposed that children and infants internalise these attachments and use them when relating to others as they grow and develop. They shape the person's personality, as well as the emotional and behavioural responses to attachment figures (Bowlby, 1973).

Building on this, Mary Ainsworth (1978) developed the strange situation experiment to test for different types of attachments. Children who were classed as having a secure attachment would demonstrate their distress initially but then return to calm when reunited with their parent. They had a parent or caregiver who could soothe and calm them after a period of separation, whereas those who did not were classed as insecure. From this finding, Ainsworth divided insecure attachment into two distinct types: avoidant and anxious/ambivalent.

Children with avoidant attachment styles tend to have parents or caregivers who are detached and prefer their children to be more independent. These children learn to 'down-regulate' and be with their own emotions, showing little or no emotional reaction to their mother leaving and returning. Those with anxious/ambivalent attachment styles usually have parents who are difficult to predict. They tend to switch from overly protective and lovable to distant and cold, ignoring the child's needs. These children usually display extreme distress in response to the separation and then become ambivalent when reunited. Main and Solomon (1990) later identified a fourth category referred to as disorganised/disoriented, in which the child seemed fearful, disorganised, confused and would freeze in the presence of the parent. This is consistent with a lack of a clear attachment style and is more commonly found in those who have been abused.

Although first developed to understand children's interactions with their caregivers, these attachment templates have been shown to be influential over the lifespan and in later developmental stages such as adulthood (Cassidy & Shaver, 1999). When attachments are disrupted in the early stages, they can affect relationships later, with the impact of extreme distress, making some people unable to form emotional bonds with others or show concern for them. This makes them more susceptible to aggression and offending behaviour (Bowlby, 1973).

In relation to this, Hirschi's (1969) social-control theory of offending behaviour proposed that offending occurs in people who do not have a secure attachment base because they have not internalised the expected social norms that help them conform to normative societal behaviour like those with a secure attachment do. Offenders have been shown to have fewer secure attachments than non-offenders (Ogilvie et al., 2014), and different types of attachment moderate the internalisation of behavioural problems (Hoeve et al., 2012), suggesting the need for skills that help them learn how to improve their distress tolerance and regulate their emotions. While it should be treated as one part of the whole picture, attachment theory is critical for explaining offending behaviour and understanding the impact of early experiences for those who are justice experienced. It can help with the development and modelling of the emotional regulation system to aid soothing and self-compassion. Interventions should target attachments and the long-term mediating impact of ACEs on the person who has offended and create the foundations for a secure base through compassion-based interventions.

Each of these theories offers valuable insights into the factors contributing to criminal behaviour, from early childhood experiences to cognitive processes, decision-making, personality traits and attachment styles. However, they also have limitations, such as deterministic views, cultural biases and an overemphasis on individual factors at the expense of social and environmental influences. A holistic understanding of criminal behaviour necessitates integrating these perspectives, recognising the potential for change and the complex interplay of various factors throughout an individual's life.

SOCIOLOGICAL

Sociological theories of offender behaviour are more interested in external factors such as the relationship between the person who offends, their family, peer groups and environmental influences.

THE THEORY OF SOCIAL DISORGANISATION

The Theory of Social Disorganisation, also known as the ecological perspective, or Chicago School Theory (Shaw & McKay, 1942), proposes that offending behaviour is more prevalent in areas with fewer socio-economic opportunities, high rates of unemployment, poor health, poor housing and more residents who have moved in and out of the community. The problem of not having a stable community is that its residents cannot come together to tackle offending in their neighbourhood, and thus, they become disorganised, allowing older criminals to organise the youth and teach them criminal behaviours. This then creates sub-cultures within the community. Contemporary theories of offending behaviour refer to the crime, place and space theory, including the 'Broken Window Theory', which explores the link between disorder and crime, 'Defensible Space Theory', which looks at the relationship between architecture and offending behaviour, and 'Routine Activities Theory'. All consider the social environment and how it can influence criminal behaviour. When considering these factors associated with offending behaviour, there are clear links between them and social/community capital that must be considered.

STRAIN AND SUB-CULTURAL THEORY

Strain Theory (Agnew, 1992) argues that crime is a consequence of the strain between goals such as status and wealth, and the means to achieve them, for example, employment and education. Strain can also come in the form of the death of a loved one or valued possession (loss of positive stimuli) or verbal or physical abuse (presentation of negative stimuli). Strain can cause the person to feel distress, anger, frustration, fear or threat and turn to offending to cope. There are disparities between the rich and the poor, which serve to increase the gap and strain on acquiring goals, and this leads to feelings of deprivation and hopelessness. When someone is unable to achieve monetary or status goals due to regular means, they will turn to offending. They may also seek revenge against their abuser or take illicit drugs to avoid hurt and feel good. This relates to Sub-Cultural Theory, where people will conform to the values and norms of a group they belong to, and in lower class young people, this usually results in offending due to their efforts to achieve social status. However, there are limitations to this theory because not all young working-class people turn to offending to alleviate status frustration.

Non-offender coping may help reduce re-offending by teaching individuals the skills of compassion. This can help them manage their emotions and distress tolerance in relation to their experience of strains. At the foundation of strain theory lies the simple truth that if people are treated harshly, they can become upset, angry and frustrated and respond in ways conducive to offending behaviour to reduce strain. It therefore makes sense that if they are treated with compassion and direct it to the self, they may respond differently, be guided towards pro-social goals, and avoid offending altogether.

SOCIAL CONTROL THEORY

Social Control Theory is more concerned with why people obey the law rather than break it. This theory was first proposed by Hirschi (1969) to understand offending behaviour by exploring what happens when someone does not conform to the social norms that help bond them to society. According to this theory, four social bonds keep people from offending. Attachment to others is measured by the strength of the bond someone has with others and their expectation of them to conform to social norms. Commitment to goals and lifestyles that fit in with the conventional norms of society and involvement in pro-social behaviours restricts the time spent engaging in offending behaviour. Belief is concerned with the person's upbringing and if they have been socialised to believe that it is the norm to abide by the law. The stronger the social bonds, the more likely someone will not offend. If these social bonds are weaker, the person will have more freedom to engage in offending. However, this model is unsupported by the lack of empirical evidence for its effectiveness.

Each theory is valuable but can be criticised for overlooking individual factors such as personal choice, psychological traits and family dynamics. They assume that all individuals in disorganised areas are equally likely to commit crimes. It does not account for changes in neighbourhoods over time or the ability of communities to develop resilience or the positive social networks and sub-cultures that can emerge in these areas. Some primarily focus on economic-related crimes and do not fully explain crimes of passion, violence or deviance that do not stem from economic strain. They assume that everyone aspires to the same goals such as acquiring wealth, overlooking diversity in individual aspirations and the complexity of human motivation. The Strain and Sub-Cultural theories focus mainly on the lower socio-economic strata, potentially overlooking strain and sub-cultural formation in middle or upper classes. With the Social Control Theory, there is an assumption that conformity is always desirable and that strong social bonds are inherently good, neglecting cases where such bonds may reinforce harmful or deviant norms. It tends to portray individuals as passively influenced by their social bonds, underestimating personal agency and the capacity for individuals to resist social pressures, and fails to explain why people commit crime and less insight into the motivations of those who break the law despite having strong social bonds.

CONCLUSION

The reasons why people offend vary widely and include factors such as a person's biology, social influences and social relationships, parenting and attachment, societal boundaries, how compassionate or empathetic they are, experiences of trauma, poverty, education and employment opportunities, social deprivation, plus issues with drugs and alcohol, and how all this impacts on mental health. All these factors should be considered when seeking to understand the causes of criminal behaviour and the interventions that aim to address the underlying issues with offending. The reasons why people offend have their roots in the biological, psychological and social. As such, desistance-focused interventions should be developed to address the bio-psychosocial causes of offending. Emotional regulation and the ability to regulate emotions feature to some degree in all the theories presented here. It would, therefore, make sense that learning to regulate emotions would be a key proponent of approaches and models to reduce offending behaviour.

Furthermore, if we are to truly understand why people offend and how we can prevent it, there is a need to consider the person's past experiences, including ACEs, their present situation, current wants or needs and their future aspirations and goals for desisting. In the next chapter, we will explore the current models of offender rehabilitation and see how they approach offences and what they do to prevent them from reoccurring.

REFERENCES

Agnew, R. (1992). Foundation for a general strain theory of crime and delinquency. *Criminology, 30*(1), 47–88.

Ainsworth, M. D. S. (1978). The Bowlby Ainsworth attachment theory. *Behavioural and Brain Sciences, 1*(3), 436–438.

Andrews, D. A., Bonta, J., & Wormith, J. S. (2006). The recent past and near future at risk and/or need assessment. *Crime & Delinquency, 52*(1), 7–17.

Astridge, B., Li, W. W., McDermott, B., & Longhitano, C. (2023). A systematic review and meta-analysis on adverse childhood experiences: Prevalence in youth offenders and their effects on youth recidivism. *Child Abuse & Neglect, 140*, 106055.

Baker, L. A., Bezdjian, S., & Raine, A. (2006). Behavioral genetics: The science of antisocial behavior. *Law and Contemporary Problems, 69*(1–2), 7.

Banse, R., Koppehele-Gossel, J., Kistemaker, L. M., Werner, V. A., & Schmidt, A. F. (2013). Pro-criminal attitudes, intervention, and recidivism. *Aggression and Violent Behavior, 18*(6), 673–685.

Bowlby, J. (1958). The nature of the child's tie to his mother. *International Journal of Psycho-Analysis, 39*, 350–373.

Bowlby, J. (1973). *Attachment and loss: Vol. 2. Separation: Anxiety and anger*. Basic Books.

Bowlby, J. (1988). *A secure base*. Basic Books.

Cassidy, J., & Shaver, P. R. (Eds.) (1999). *Handbook of attachment: Theory, research, and clinical applications*. Rough Guides.

Choy, O., Portnoy, J., Raine, A., Remmel, R., Schug, R., Tuvblad, C., & Yang, Y. (2018). Biological influences on offending across the life course. In D. Farrington, L. Kazemian, & A. Piquero (Eds.), *The Oxford handbook of developmental and life-course criminology* (pp. 325–354). Oxford University Press.

Cornish, D. B., & Clarke, R. V. (1987). Understanding crime displacement: An application of rational choice theory. *Criminology, 25*(4), 933–948.

Craig, J. M., Piquero, A. R., Farrington, D. P., & Ttofi, M. M. (2017). A little early risk goes a long bad way: Adverse childhood experiences and life-course offending in the Cambridge study. *Journal of Criminal Justice, 53*, 34–45.

da Cunha-Bang, S., Fisher, P. M., Hjordt, L. V., Perfalk, E., Persson Skibsted, A., Bock, C., Ohlhues Baandrup, A., Deen, M., Thomsen, C., Sestoft, D. M., & Knudsen, G. M. (2017). Violent offenders respond to provocations with high amygdala and striatal reactivity. *Social Cognitive and Affective Neuroscience, 12*(5), 802–810. https://doi.org/10.1093/scan/nsx006

Davis, M. H. (1983). Measuring individual differences in empathy: Evidence for a multidimensional approach. *Journal of Personality and Social Psychology, 44*(1), 113.

De Looff, P. C., Cornet, L. J., De Kogel, C. H., Fernández-Castilla, B., Embregts, P. J., Didden, R., & Nijman, H. L. (2022). Heart rate and skin conductance associations with physical aggression, psychopathy, antisocial personality disorder and conduct disorder: An updated meta-analysis. *Neuroscience & Biobehavioral Reviews, 132*, 553–582.

Ellis, L., & Hoskin, A. W. (2015). The evolutionary neuroandrogenic theory of criminal behavior expanded. *Aggression and Violent Behavior, 24*, 61–74.

Facer-Irwin, E., Karatzias, T., Bird, A., Blackwood, N., & MacManus, D. (2022). PTSD and complex PTSD in sentenced male prisoners in the UK: Prevalence, trauma antecedents, and psychiatric comorbidities. *Psychological Medicine, 52*(13), 2794–2804.

Felitti, V. J., Anda, R. F., Nordenberg, D., Williamson, D. F., Spitz, A. M., Edwards, V., Koss, M. P., & Marks, J. S. (1998). Relationship of childhood abuse and household dysfunction to many of the leading causes of death in adults. *American Journal of Preventive Medicine, 14*(4), 245–258.

Gao, Y., Tuvblad, C., Schell, A., Baker, L., & Raine, A. (2015). Skin conductance fear conditioning impairments and aggression: A longitudinal study. *Psychophysiology, 52*(2), 288–295.

Garbutt, K., Rennoldson, M., & Gregson, M. (2023). Shame and self-compassion connect childhood experience of adversity with harm inflicted on the self and others. *Journal of Interpersonal Violence, 38*(11–12), 7193–7214.

Gard, A. M., Dotterer, H. L., & Hyde, L. W. (2019). Genetic influences on antisocial behavior: Recent advances and future directions. *Current Opinion in Psychology, 27*, 46–55.

Geurts, D. E., Von Borries, K., Volman, I., Bulten, B. H., Cools, R., & Verkes, R. J. (2016). Neural connectivity during reward expectation dissociates psychopathic criminals from non-criminal individuals with high impulsive/antisocial psychopathic traits. *Social Cognitive and Affective Neuroscience, 11*(8), 1326–1334.

Gilbert, P. (2007). The evolution of shame as a marker for relationship security: A biopsychosocial approach. In J. L. Tracy, R. W. Robins, & J. P. Tangney (Eds.), *The self-conscious emotions: Theory and research* (pp. 283–309). The Guilford Press.

Gilbert, P. (2009). Introducing compassion-focused therapy. *Advances in Psychiatric Treatment, 15*(3), 199–208.

Gilbert, P. (2017). Exploring compassion focused therapy in forensic settings: An evolutionary and social-contextual approach. In J. Davies & C. Nagi (Eds.), *Individual psychological therapies in forensic settings* (pp. 59–84). Routledge.

Glenn, A. L., & Raine, A. (2014). Neurocriminology: Implications for the punishment, prediction and prevention of criminal behaviour. *Nature Reviews Neuroscience, 15*(1), 54–63.

Glenn, A. L., & Yang, Y. (2012). The potential role of the striatum in antisocial behavior and psychopathy. *Biological Psychiatry, 72*(10), 817–822.

Hare, R. D. (2003). *The Hare psychopathy checklist-revised* (2nd ed.). Multi-Health Syst.

Hirschi, T. (1969). *Causes of delinquency*. University of California Press.

Hoeve, M., Stams, G. J. J., Van der Put, C. E., Dubas, J. S., Van der Laan, P. H., & Gerris, J. R. (2012). A meta-analysis of attachment to parents and delinquency. *Journal of Abnormal Child Psychology, 40*, 771–785.

Jolliffe, D., & Farrington, D. P. (2024). The promotive relationship between personality and self-reported offending. *Psychology, Crime and Law*, *30*(4), 319–337.

Jump, D., & Gray, P. (2024). Partners in crime: Integrating forensic psychotherapy into criminological discourse. *The International Journal of Forensic Psychotherapy*, *6*(1), 86–99.

Kohlberg, L. (1971). *Stages of moral development as a basis for moral education*. Center for Moral Education, Harvard University.

Ling, S., & Raine, A. (2018). The neuroscience of psychopathy and forensic implications. *Psychology, Crime and Law*, *24*(3), 296–312.

Ling, S., Umbach, R., & Raine, A. (2019). Biological explanations of criminal behavior. *Psychology, Crime and Law*, *25*(6), 626–640.

Lombroso, C. (1876). *L'Uomo delinquente*. Hoepli.

Main, M., & Solomon, J. (1990). Procedures for identifying infants as disorganized/disoriented during the Ainsworth Strange Situation. In M. T. Greenberg, D. Cicchetti, & E. M. Cummings (Eds.), *Attachment in the preschool years: Theory, research, and intervention* (pp. 121–160). The University of Chicago Press.

Malvaso, C. G., Cale, J., Whitten, T., Day, A., Singh, S., Hackett, L., Delfabbro, P. H., & Ross, S. (2022). Associations between adverse childhood experiences and trauma among young people who offend: A systematic literature review. *Trauma, Violence, & Abuse*, *23*(5), 1677–1694. https://doi.org/10.1177/15248380211013132

Martí-Vilar, M., Serrano-Pastor, L., & Sala, F. G. (2019). Emotional, cultural, and cognitive variables of prosocial behaviour. *Current Psychology*, *38*, 912–919.

Maruna, S. (2004). Desistance from crime and explanatory style: A new direction in the psychology of reform. *Journal of Contemporary Criminal Justice*, *20*(2), 184–200.

Maruna, S., & Copes, H. (2005). What have we learned from five decades of neutralization research? *Crime and Justice*, *32*, 221–320.

Maruna, S., & Mann, R. E. (2006). A fundamental attribution error? Rethinking cognitive distortions. *Legal and Criminological Psychology*, *11*(2), 155–177.

Meijers, J., Harte, J. M., Meynen, G., & Cuijpers, P. (2017). Differences in executive functioning between violent and non-violent offenders. *Psychological Medicine, 47*(10), 1784–1793.

Miller, J. D., & Lynam, D. R. (2003). Psychopathy and the five-factor model of personality: A replication and extension. *Journal of Personality Assessment, 81*(2), 168–178.

Ó'Ciardha, C., & Ward, T. (2013). Theories of cognitive distortions in sexual offending: What the current research tells us. *Trauma, Violence, & Abuse, 14*(1), 5–21.

Ogilvie, C. A., Newman, E., Todd, L., & Peck, D. (2014). Attachment & violent offending: A meta-analysis. *Aggression and Violent Behavior, 19*(4), 322–339.

Raine, A. (2002). The biological basis of crime. *Crime: Public Policies for Crime Control, 43*, 74.

Raine, A., & Yang, Y. (2006). Neural foundations to moral reasoning and antisocial behavior. *Social Cognitive and Affective Neuroscience, 1*(3), 203–213.

Reavis, J. A., Looman, J., Franco, K. A., & Rojas, B. (2013). Adverse childhood experiences and adult criminality: How long must we live before we possess our own lives? *The Permanente Journal, 17*(2), 44.

Roberts, B. W., Luo, J., Briley, D. A., Chow, P. I., Su, R., & Hill, P. L. (2017). A systematic review of personality trait change through intervention. *Psychological Bulletin, 143*(2), 117.

Sajadian, M., Younesi, S. J., Jafari, P., Azkhosh, M., Yarandi, R. B., & Kordbagheri, M. (2024). Shame, fear of compassion, self-criticism, and self-reassurance mediate the effect of early life events on emotional disorders among male prisoners: A structural equation modelling analysis. *Acta Psychologica, 242*, 104116.

Sapolsky, R. M. (2004). The frontal cortex and the criminal justice system. *Philosophical Transactions of the Royal Society B: Biological Sciences, 359*(1451), 1787.

Seligman, M. E. P., & Elder, G. H. (1986). Explanatory style across the life span: Achievement and health. In A. Sorenson, F. E. Weinert, & L. Sherrod (Eds.), *Learned helplessness and life span development* (pp. 377–427). Erlbaum.

Shaw, C. R., & McKay, H. D. (1942). *Juvenile delinquency and urban areas*. University of Chicago Press.

Sousa, R., Petrocchi, N., Gilbert, P., & Rijo, D. (2022). Unveiling the heart of young offenders: Testing the tripartite model of affect regulation in community and forensic male adolescents. *Journal of Criminal Justice*, *82*, 101970.

Sutherland, E. H. (1934, 1939, 1947). *Principles of criminology* (3rd ed.). Lippincott.

Svingen, E. (2023). PTSD and crime propensity: Stress systems, brain structures, and the nature of the relationship. *Heliyon*, *7*(9), e18381.

Tharshini, N. K., Ibrahim, F., Kamaluddin, M. R., Rathakrishnan, B., & Che Mohd Nasir, N. (2021). The link between individual personality traits and criminality: A systematic review. *International Journal of Environmental Research and Public Health*, *18*(16), 8663.

Turner, D., Wolf, A. J., Barra, S., Müller, M., Gregório Hertz, P., Huss, M., Tüscher, O., & Retz, W. (2021). The association between adverse childhood experiences and mental health problems in young offenders. *European Child & Adolescent Psychiatry*, *30*(8), 1195–1207. https://doi.org/10.1007/s00787-020-01608-2

Van Vugt, E., Hendriks, J., Stams, G. J., Van Exter, F., Bijleveld, C., Van der Laan, P., & Asscher, J. (2011). Moral judgment, cognitive distortions and implicit theories in young sex offenders. *Journal of Forensic Psychiatry and Psychology*, *22*(4), 603–619.

Walters, G. D. (1995). The psychological inventory of criminal thinking styles: Part I: Reliability and preliminary validity. *Criminal Justice and Behavior*, *22*(3), 307–325.

Walters, G. D. (2006). Use of the Psychological Inventory of Criminal Thinking Styles to predict disciplinary adjustment in male inmate program participants. *International Journal of Offender Therapy and Comparative Criminology*, *50*(2), 166–173.

Wright, E. M., & Schwartz, J. A. (2021). The influence of adverse childhood experiences on internalizing and externalizing problems in early adulthood: Evidence of a gene× environment× sex interaction. *Child Abuse & Neglect*, *114*, 104962.

Yang, Y., Narr, K. L., Baker, L. A., Joshi, S. H., Jahanshad, N., Raine, A., & Thompson, P. M. (2015). Frontal and striatal alterations associated with psychopathic traits in adolescents. *Psychiatry Research: Neuroimaging*, *231*(3), 333–340.

Zannas, A. S., Provençal, N., & Binder, E. B. (2015). Epigenetics of posttraumatic stress disorder: Current evidence, challenges, and future directions. *Biological Psychiatry*, *78*(5), 327–335.

Zeng, Y., Liu, X., & Cheng, L. (2022). Facial emotion perceptual tendency in violent and non-violent offenders. *Journal of Interpersonal Violence*, *37*(17–18), NP15058–NP15074.

Zhao, J., Wang, X., Zhang, H., & Zhao, R. (2021). Rational choice theory applied to an explanation of juvenile offender decision making in the Chinese setting. *International Journal of Offender Therapy and Comparative Criminology*, *65*(4), 434–457.

3

CURRENT MODELS FOR THE REHABILITATION AND PREVENTION OF OFFENDING BEHAVIOUR

ABSTRACT

This chapter shifts focus from the underlying causes of offending to current rehabilitation approaches and models. It begins with an overview of the rehabilitation movement, emphasising the principle of 'what works' in offender reform. The discussion then moves on to explore two major frameworks: the Risk-Need-Responsivity (RNR) model and the Good Lives Model (GLM). Each model will be briefly outlined and critically evaluated for its effectiveness in preventing re-offending and supporting desistance. The chapter concludes with a rationale for introducing a new approach to rehabilitation, the Compassionate Positive Applied Strengths-based Solutions (COMPASS) model, summarising its potential benefits for enhancing desistance support.

Keywords: RNR; risks; strengths; GLM; rehabilitation; interventions

REHABILITATION OF OFFENDERS AND THE PREVENTION OF OFFENDING BEHAVIOUR

Historically, rehabilitation was viewed as a form of repentance for sins, with prison serving as a place for reflection and behaviour change. This perspective shifted in the 20th century towards a more scientific and medical approach, treating offending behaviours as flaws that could be addressed through intervention. Evolutionarily, rehabilitation can be seen as a form of forgiveness that influences a person's acceptance and rejection within their social group

(Ward et al., 2022). The modern 'what works' movement, initiated by Martinson's (1974) controversial assertion that 'nothing works' in offender rehabilitation, sparked a shift in focus. Despite his claim, it became clear that incarceration alone was ineffective at reducing re-offending rates. This led to a renewed emphasis on interventions and alternative approaches to support rehabilitation and reduce recidivism (Bonta & Andrews, 2016). Consequently, guidelines were established based on principles of intensity, responsivity and learning style, often using Cognitive Behavioural Therapy (CBT) methods (Andrews & Bonta, 2003). In the United Kingdom, rehabilitation pro-grammes, such as Enhanced Thinking Skills (ETS) and its successor, the Thinking Skills Programme (TSP), were developed to address offending behaviour (Hollin & Palmer, 2009). However, these programmes have had mixed results, with high dropout rates and continued re-offending among some participants. The 'what works' approach, which relies heavily on experimental research and randomised controlled trials, often overlooks the personal experiences and future aspirations of offenders. Critics argue that these models focus more on community safety than on understanding and addressing the root causes of offending behaviour (Ward & Maruna, 2007). A growing perspective suggests that both 'what works' and 'what helps' should be considered. By understanding the individual needs and experiences of those who have desisted from offending, practitioners can better support others in their journey towards rehabilitation. Rehabilitation, therefore, is not only a political and personal goal but also a collaborative process where the person's own experiences and needs are central to effective intervention, making the audience feel included and part of the solution. This chapter will explore two dominant models of offender rehabilitation – Risk-Need-Responsivity (RNR) and the Good Lives Model (GLM), highlighting their strengths and limitations in preventing offending and supporting desistance.

THE TWO MODELS OF OFFENDER REHABILITATION

Here, we will briefly explore the two main models of offender rehabilitation: The RNR and the GLM. The two models are the most current and widely used ways of working with people who have offended, with one focused on risk management (RNR) and the other on strengths-based approaches to rehabil-itation. An overview is provided for each model as well as some of the gaps and limitations of both.

THE RNR MODEL

Based on the social learning and personality theory of criminal behaviour, the RNR model is arguably the most influential and globally successful model for assessing and treating offending behaviour. First published in 1990 by Andrews, Bonta and Hodge, the RNR model outlined three principles, risk, need and responsivity, that are associated with the effective assessment and treatment of offenders. This model is heavily invested in the medical/therapeutic approach to offending behaviour and sees offending as being based on deficits of character and behaviour. From the Risk/Need principle, the RNR model assumes that all offender behaviour is the outcome of socially learned behaviours, and the risks and rewards of offending are weighed against the benefits of pro-social behaviour (Bonta & Andrews, 2007).

Risk

The Risk principle is concerned with matching the intervention intensity to the level of risk, with higher risk associated with programmes of greater intensity. It assumes that criminal behaviour could be predicted, and interventions targeted to higher risk offenders. The Risk principle contains two parts. One relates to the assessment of risk and how offenders can be split into high, medium and low-risk offender groups. The other explains the level of treatment given to the person in response to their offending. Assessment of risks are undertaken using tried and tested measures such as the HCR-20 (Webster et al., 1997). These measures focus on the presence of risks, their relevance to the individuals offending and strategies that can be used to mitigate risk (Douglas & Reeves, 2010).

Need

The Need principle focuses on the criminogenic needs of offenders that lead to or put them at risk of offending. Its goal is to match the treatment intervention to the criminogenic needs and the risk factors associated with offending behaviour that Andrews and Bonta (2003) refer to as the dynamic or central eight risk factors. They are:

(1) History of anti-social behaviour.

(2) Anti-social personality pattern.

(3) Anti-social/pro-criminal attitudes.

(4) Anti-social associates.

(5) Problematic circumstances at home (family/marital relationships).

(6) Problematic circumstances at work/school.

(7) Few/no pro-social recreation activities.

(8) Substance abuse.

It also includes four 'minor' needs:

(1) Self-esteem.

(2) Vague feelings of personal distress.

(3) Major mental disorder such as psychosis or personality disorder.

(4) Physical health.

Using mainly CBT techniques-based interventions, the goal of RNR is to turn these needs into non-criminal ones. For example, turning pro-criminal attitudes into pro-social ones or addressing anti-social personality patterns and aggression with anger management courses and self-management skills. Self-esteem, mental health and distress are considered minor in the RNR model despite data from a recent meta-analysis revealing them to be important predictors of offending behaviour (Basto-Pereira & Farrington, 2022).

Responsivity

The Responsivity principle explains how the intervention should be delivered and matched to the person's learning style and ability. It suggests that all behaviour can be addressed through cognitive social learning interventions. Responsivity is split into general and specific. General responsivity works in two ways; one is based on the principle of developing a warm, collaborative, respectful and sup-portive relationship with the client, while the other (the structuring principle) is concerned with directing behaviour change through modelling, problem-solving and reinforcement. Specific responsivity focuses on socio-biological personality factors and the person's individual strengths that can help or hinder offender treatment. This responsivity is about the personal factors of an individual that can enhance their treatment. Although responsivity utilises personal strengths, it does so to reduce recidivism rather than with a focus on the person's goals and aims for a crime-free future.

RNR Interventions and How They Attempt to Change Offending Behaviour

The RNR model tends to implement CBT-based interventions in its rehabilitation of offenders. CBT is one of the most widely used forms of offender treatment for reducing recidivism. The underlying premise of this approach is that criminal thinking is a learned rather than innate cognitive deficit, and that therapy works by challenging maladaptive patterns of thinking that contribute to emotional and behavioural issues related to criminal thinking and behaviour (Yates, 2013). Common distorted cognitive thinking styles include schemas of entitlement and dominance, supplanting blame, immoral reasoning, misreading social cues and self-justification thinking (Beck & Freeman, 1990). This type of criminal thinking can lead to non-threatening situations being viewed as threatening or them considering themselves to be the victim who is shunned or not given a chance by society (Lipsey et al., 2007).

CBT is an effective therapeutic strategy for reducing recidivism among medium- and high-risk offenders (Kosson et al., 2019). Research suggests that CBT is effective for anger management, cognitive skills training, relapse prevention and moral development and has been found to reduce the risk of re-offending by 23% for general offending and 28% for violent offending (Henwood et al., 2015; Lipsey et al., 2007). There are several different CBT programmes, such as Thinking for a Change (Bush et al., 1997), Moral Recognition Therapy (Little & Robinson, 1988) and Aggression Replacement Training (Glick & Goldstein, 1987), and more that have been developed for offenders. These programmes teach people about accountability and how thinking, attitudes and choices led to their criminal behaviour. CBT techniques help the person identify cognitive deficits and faulty thinking styles that can be addressed through the restructuring of maladaptive cognitive biases (Lipsey et al., 2007) and the improvement of morality.

Limitations of the RNR Model

The RNR model, despite its widespread use in offender rehabilitation, has several significant limitations:

Age differences and effectiveness: CBT, a cornerstone of RNR interventions, has shown varying levels of effectiveness depending on the age of the offenders. Research indicates that CBT is less effective for high-risk adult offenders compared to younger offenders, aligning with Sampson and Laub's (2003) Life Course Theory (Han et al., 2023). Moral Recognition Therapy, initially deemed effective for adults, has been found to be less effective for youth offenders and no more effective for adults with mental health issues than standard treatments in reducing recidivism (Blonigen et al., 2022; Heynen et al., 2023). This suggests that different therapeutic approaches, such as Compassion-Focused Therapy (CFT), might be more suitable for younger offenders (Ribeiro da Silva et al., 2021).

Lack of consideration for capital: RNR interventions often focus on cognitive and behavioural change without addressing critical social and economic factors influencing desistance, such as housing, employment and financial stability. Beaudry et al. (2021) found limited evidence that CBT-based programmes reduce re-offending risk in prison settings. The effectiveness of these programmes is higher in community settings, highlighting the need for comprehensive support that addresses both criminal behaviour and post-release reintegration challenges (Lipsey et al., 2007).

Issues with transition and resettlement: Inadequate resettlement programmes, such as the United Kingdom's 'Through the Gate' initiative, fail to effectively assess and address the resettlement needs of prisoners, impacting their transition back into the community (HMI Probation, 2017). Effective rehabilitation requires that release plans consider criminogenic risks, future goals and psychosocial needs from the start of sentencing and are continuously reviewed throughout incarceration and after release.

Blaming the individual: CBT and RNR approaches have been criticised for potentially blaming individuals for their criminal thinking (Morse et al., 2022). These models often adopt a 'fix what is wrong' approach rather than an 'understand what is wrong' approach. This focus on altering thinking patterns neglects deeper emotional issues and past experiences, such as Adverse Childhood Experiences (ACEs), which can be pivotal in understanding and addressing criminal behaviour. Confrontational approaches are less effective than those incorporating empathy, encouragement and warmth, such as CFT (Gilbert, 2009).

Lower effectiveness outside laboratory settings: While meta-analyses show RNR principles can reduce re-offending among violent, general and sex offenders (Bonta et al., 2014; Dowden & Andrews, 1999; Hanson et al., 2009), real-world applications of these programmes have lower mean effect sizes (Bonta & Andrews, 2016). Studies indicate that RNR interventions may be no more effective than control interventions in reducing recidivism (Seewald et al., 2018), suggesting that rigid adherence to RNR principles may not be necessary for effective desistance support in the community (Duan et al., 2024).

Questionable evidence for Risk principle: A review by Fazel et al. (2024) found that evidence supporting the Risk principle of the RNR model is low, with non-significant effect sizes and potential author biases influencing outcomes. This calls into question the validity and reliability of the RNR model in evaluating and rehabilitating offenders within the justice system. In their narrative review, Challinor et al. (2021) found no empirical evidence that the HCR-20 was effective at reducing violence, with Vojt et al. (2013) suggesting that it does not predict future violence. Furthermore, despite the effectiveness of the HCR-20, it is more concerned with the risk factors of offending and less about the human being behind the offence.

While the RNR model has shown some success in reducing recidivism, it faces significant limitations related to age differences, lack of consideration for socio-economic factors, inadequate resettlement support, potential individual blaming, lower real-world effectiveness and questionable evidence for its Risk principle. The GLM was introduced in 2000 as an alternative and complementary approach to the RNR.

THE GOOD LIVES MODEL

The GLM was developed in response to the limitations of the RNR model, mainly the one-sided and arguably negative focus on risks. Ward et al. (2012) proposed that the RNR model failed to consider a person's needs and possibilities of living what they refer to as a good life. This model was originally developed for sex offenders but has now been applied to other offender groups. Taking inspiration from positive psychology and strengths-based approaches, from the GLM perspective, criminal behaviour is understood as a maladaptive means of achieving needs and goals in life. This model assumes that offenders want the same things as non-offenders but go about getting them through anti-social ways. The GLM model refers to things people want and categorises them into 11 primary human goods:

(1) Life (healthy living and functioning).

(2) Knowledge (being informed about things that are important to them).

(3) Excellence in play (hobbies and recreational pursuits).

(4) Excellence in work (including mastery experiences).

(5) Excellence in agency (autonomy and self-directedness).

(6) Inner peace (freedom from emotional turmoil and stress).

(7) Relatedness (including intimate, romantic and familial relationships).

(8) Community (connection to wider social groups).

(9) Spirituality (in the broad sense of finding meaning and purpose in life).

(10) Pleasure (the state of happiness or feeling good in the here and now).

(11) Creativity (expressing oneself through alternative forms).

Secondary goods are the activities and means by which someone seeks to achieve primary goods or goals. For example, someone whose goal is the good of relatedness would seek out pro-social friendships and peer groups or a loving relationship with the opposite sex rather than commit a sexual offence to acquire the good. Secondary goods can be considered the same as criminogenic risk factors when they create barriers to reaching goals through non-harmful means (Willis et al., 2013).

The GLM model identifies two types of problems that can occur when someone is pursuing their life goals: internal and external capacities. Internal capacities are the psychological, cognitive and behavioural capacities, and external capacities are the factors that can support non-offending such as employment or support. The opposite of these same factors can also be considered risks to offending. The GLM has two routes into offending. One is the direct route, where people actively engage in offending behaviour, and the other is the indirect route, where they do so through unintended ways, such as becoming aggressive after consuming alcohol or substances and attacking others. This can help guide practitioners towards the most suitable intervention for the person who has offended.

GLM Interventions and How They Aim to Change Offending Behaviour

The GLM uses interventions that help a person identify their primary goods and develop the skills and attitudes to achieve them through non-criminal means (Willis & Ward, 2013). Working with the offender, they develop an individualised good life plan and explore ways of reaching goals that contribute to that person's good life, rather than a one-size-fits-all approach.

Even though risks are acknowledged, more attention is given to what can help increase well-being. Group therapy and motivational interviewing are two methods used in the GLM (Harkins et al., 2012). GLM interventions include CBT and social learning techniques to reduce the risk of offending, in addition to empathy training, emotional regulation and social skills training to develop the internal capacities that support the goal of acquiring primary good through non-criminal behaviour (Willis & Ward, 2013).

The interventions are facilitated by a positive, empathic, warm and encouraging practitioner who guides the person throughout with set tasks and homework assignments that can be completed in between sessions. Clients are encouraged to surround themselves with pro-social others who can keep the person on the 'straight and narrow' and help them achieve their goals. A Good Lives Plan (GLP) is developed with the client that sets out their plans to reach their goals and is revised or updated during each session (Ward & Gannon, 2006). The plan involves exploring risks and what they want to achieve from their offending. This is then used to explore alternative routes to that goal without the criminal involvement in offending behaviours. In addition to this, their support systems and work/education options upon release are discussed, and any concerns are implemented into the plan. The GLP is an individualised plan for what that person needs going forward. Treatment time varies and depends on the client's engagement and responsivity to the interventions (Ward & Gannon, 2006).

Limitations of the GLM

The GLM offers a positive approach to offender rehabilitation, yet several limitations challenge its effectiveness and applicability:

Lack of Empirical Support: Despite its theoretical appeal, the GLM lacks robust empirical support. Bonta and Andrews (2003) and Ogloff and Davis (2004) have pointed out that the model has not been sufficiently validated through empirical studies. Most research evaluating the GLM has focused on sexual offenders, raising concerns about its external validity when applied to a broader offender population (Yates, 2013). A recent literature review by Zeccola et al. (2021) found insufficient evidence to suggest that the GLM effectively reduces recidivism across all offender types. The review noted the limited number of studies meeting inclusion criteria, with most involving sex offenders and few demonstrating that GLM approaches could sustain motivation for desistance.

Stigma and Disengagement: The GLM's origins in treating sex offenders present a significant barrier to its broader application. The stigma associated with sex offenders can lead to disengagement from the model by other offender groups. Additionally, the idea of promoting a 'good life' for offenders can be contentious, as segments of society may feel that certain offenders, particularly sex offenders, do not deserve such goals.

Use of CBT: While the GLM incorporates CBT techniques, it faces similar limitations to traditional CBT approaches, which is that it may not be suitable for all individuals. Taylor and Hocken (2021) note that developing empathy, problem-solving skills and behavioural reflection depends heavily on the individual's motivation. Empathy, for instance, can be manipulated for anti-social purposes if not coupled with compassionate motivation. An empathic torturer, for example, may exploit their understanding of suffering to inflict greater harm, highlighting the potential misuse of empathy without compassionate intent.

Ambiguous strengths-based approach: The GLM is described as a strengths-based model, but the distinction between strengths and goods is often unclear. Strengths are the means to achieve goods, yet the model does not specify what strengths are necessary for attaining these goods and life goals. Willis and Ward (2013) argue that the GLM functions more as a framework guiding practitioners rather than a concrete method of rehabilitation.

Terminology and communication: Terminology in the GLM, such as 'excellence in work' and 'excellence in agency', can be off-putting and create barriers to desistance. These terms imply a need for high achievement, which may not align with the realistic goals of individuals seeking to reintegrate into society. Many desisting individuals may prioritise stability and routine over excellence, and the pressure to achieve high standards could lead to relapse into substance abuse or offending behaviours due to the stress of unrealistic expectations. The emphasis on 'excellence in agency' places significant responsibility for desistance on the individual, potentially overlooking the social and environmental factors influencing behaviour. This can lead to an unrealistic expectation of self-sufficiency and ignore the broader context needed for effective rehabilitation.

RATIONALE FOR A DIFFERENT APPROACH TO OFFENDING BEHAVIOUR

Lutz et al. (2022) argue that effective treatment and rehabilitation of offenders cannot rely solely on risk management or on promoting offenders' goals. Risk management models, such as the RNR model, present a pessimistic view, while models promoting offender goals, like the GLM, can be overly optimistic. The RNR model emphasises managing risks and addressing criminogenic needs but tends to overlook the individual's aspirations and goals. Conversely, the GLM adopts a humanistic approach, focusing on developing personal strengths and supporting positive goals, but it often neglects the social and environmental factors influencing offending.

A different approach is needed that integrates the importance of addressing risks and criminogenic needs with the individual's hopes and aspirations for a meaningful future. Compassion can be a crucial therapeutic bridge, linking past and present risks with future goals and facilitating desistance. However, the RNR and GLM models lack a clear vision of how compassion can support desistance. While compassion might be implied through the notion of a supportive practitioner, explicit strategies for developing and utilising compassion are not well-defined.

The RNR model's focus on deficits and risk factors fails to acknowledge the broader context of offending, including traumatic backgrounds and neurobiological factors (Taylor et al., 2020). Basto-Pereira et al. (2024) highlight how impoverished environments can exacerbate risks for youth, yet the RNR model does not adequately address these social and environmental influences. Although the GLM acknowledges the importance of social conditions upon re-entry, it provides limited guidance on how to support offenders during these transitions. The GLM's emphasis on individual agency also underestimates the impact of social and environmental factors on criminal behaviour, leaving practitioners feeling uncertain about how to apply the model effectively (Prescott & Willis, 2022). The reductionist view of offenders as merely 'criminals' in the RNR model overlooks their potential for change and the role of identity transformation in desistance (Maruna, 2001). Offenders need to be seen as individuals with potential for change rather than being defined solely by their offences or risks. Both the RNR and GLM models offer rigid frameworks that fail to fully address the complexity of offending and desistance. For instance, the GLM's broad list of primary goods and the RNR's numerous risk factors are insufficient for understanding the intricate reasons behind offending and supporting change (Polaschek, 2012).

Furthermore, the models' lack of attention to trauma and cultural context limits their effectiveness. The GLM's focus on primary goods does not account for cultural variations or the impact of past trauma. For example, autonomy as a primary good may not align with collective cultural narratives, and the models fail to address how trauma-informed care can be integrated into practice. In practice, implementing the RNR principles has proven challenging, with some practitioners opting for informal risk assessments over the rigid principles of the model (Viglione, 2019). This rigidity can hinder engagement and motivation, resulting in intervention goals that are imposed rather than collaboratively developed.

Ward et al. (2022) recommend that listening to offenders' experiences and integrating their insights can offer valuable perspectives on what causes crime and what facilitates desistance. In line with this, compassion and positive psychology, both of which have contributed to my own personal desistance from offending, should play a more prominent role. These approaches address emotional factors, such as self-esteem and distress, critical for effective intervention. Compassionate Mind Training (CMT) has been shown to be particularly beneficial for addressing shame and trauma, offering a promising alternative to traditional cognitive-behavioural therapies (Gilbert & Procter, 2006). Compassion-focused approaches can help explore past traumas and enhance responsiveness to interventions, potentially improving desistance outcomes (Taylor & Hocken, 2024). Heynen et al. (2023) suggest that future interventions should focus on self-conscious emotions like shame and guilt, advocating for CFT as a tool for both therapeutic practice and guiding practitioners. This approach, combined with positive psychology, addresses both the causes of offending and the goals of desistance, helping individuals achieve a meaningful and happy life.

CONCLUSION

Considering the many theories behind offending, neither model addresses some of the pressing issues for why people offend, or how these can be turned around to help people change their lives. Looking at the theories of why people offend in the previous chapter, it would make sense to incorporate them into the model with suggestions for addressing the issues. What is needed is a model that considers the biological, psychological and social factors that contribute to a person engaging in offending behaviours and how, by attending to these factors with compassion and positive psychology, they can be assisted when desisting from offending from the perspective of human, social, justice and community capital. Desistance from offending should consider the importance of a good life for someone aiming to stop offending and the value of a meaningful and happy life. It should be developed for and attend to the unique individual and collective capital needs of all offenders and concerning their goals explore past experiences, present situations and future aspirations to chart a course for desistance.

REFERENCES

Andrews, D. A., & Bonta, J. (2003). Prediction of criminal behavior and classification of offenders. In D. A. Andrews & J. Bonta (Eds.), *The psychology of criminal conduct* (3rd ed., pp. 185–222). Anderson Publishing Co.

Andrews, D., Bonta, J., & Hoge, R. (1990). Classification for effective rehabilitation: Rediscovering psychology. *Criminal Justice and Behavior*, *17*(1), 19–52.

Basto-Pereira, M., & Farrington, D. P. (2022). Developmental predictors of offending and persistence in crime: A systematic review of meta-analyses. *Aggression and Violent Behavior*, *65*, 101761.

Basto-Pereira, M., Farrington, D. P., & Maciel, L. (2024). Unravelling the sequences of risk factors underlying the development of criminal behavior. *Journal of Developmental and Life-Course Criminology*, 1–23.

Beaudry, G., Yu, R., Perry, A. E., & Fazel, S. (2021). Effectiveness of psychological interventions in prison to reduce recidivism: A systematic review and meta-analysis of randomised controlled trials. *The Lancet Psychiatry*, *8*(9), 759–773.

Beck, A. T., & Freeman, A. M. (1990). *Cognitive therapy of personality disorders*. Guilford Press.

Blonigen, D. M., Cucciare, M. A., Byrne, T., Shaffer, P. M., Giordano, B., Smith, J. S., Timko, C., Rosenthal, J., & Smelson, D. (2022). A randomized controlled trial of moral reconation therapy to reduce risk for criminal recidivism among justice-involved adults in mental health residential treatment. *Journal of Consulting and Clinical Psychology*, *90*(5), 413–426. https://doi.org/10.1037/ccp0000721

Bonta, J., & Andrews, D. A. (2003). A commentary on Ward and Stewart's model of human needs. *Psychology, Crime and Law*, *9*, 215–218.

Bonta, J., & Andrews, D. A. (2007). Risk-need-responsivity model for offender assessment and rehabilitation. *Rehabilitation*, *6*(1), 1–22.

Bonta, J., & Andrews, D. A. (2016). *The psychology of criminal conduct*. Routledge.

Bonta, J., Blais, J., & Wilson, H. A. (2014). A theoretically informed meta-analysis of the risk for general and violent recidivism for mentally disordered offenders. *Aggression and Violent Behavior*, *19*(3), 278–287.

Bush, J., Glick, B., & Taymans, J. (1997). *Thinking for a change*. National Institute of Corrections, United States Department of Justice.

Challinor, A., Ogundalu, A., McIntyre, J. C., Bramwell, V., & Nathan, R. (2021). The empirical evidence base for the use of the HCR-20: A narrative review of study designs and transferability of results to clinical practice. *International Journal of Law and Psychiatry, 78*, 101729. https://doi.org/10.1016/j.ijlp.2021.101729

Douglas, K. S., & Reeves, K. A. (2010). Historical-Clinical-Risk Management-20 (HCR-20) Violence Risk Assessment Scheme: Rationale, application, and empirical overview. In R. K. Otto & K. S. Douglas (Eds.), *Handbook of violence risk assessment* (pp. 147–185). Routledge/Taylor & Francis Group.

Dowden, C., & Andrews, D. A. (1999). What works for female offenders: A meta-analytic review. *Crime & Delinquency, 45*(4), 438–452.

Duan, W., Wang, Z., Yang, C., & Ke, S. (2024). Are risk-need-responsivity principles golden? A meta-analysis of randomized controlled trials of community correction programs. *Journal of Experimental Criminology, 20*(2), 593–616.

Fazel, S., Hurton, C., Burghart, M., DeLisi, M., & Yu, R. (2024). An updated evidence synthesis on the risk-need-responsivity (RNR) model: Umbrella review and commentary. *Journal of Criminal Justice, 92*, 102197.

Gilbert, P. (2009). Introducing compassion-focused therapy. *Advances in Psychiatric Treatment, 15*(3), 199–208.

Gilbert, P., & Procter, S. (2006). Compassionate mind training for people with high shame and self-criticism: Overview and pilot study of a group therapy approach. *Clinical Psychology & Psychotherapy, 13*(6), 353–379.

Glick, B., & Goldstein, A. P. (1987). Aggression replacement training. *Journal of Counseling and Development, 65*(7), 356–362.

Han, S., Piquero, A. R., & Bersani, B. E. (2023). Does rational choice help to explain offending differences across immigrant generations? Focusing on serious adolescent offenders. *Journal of Research in Crime and Delinquency, 0*(0).

Hanson, R. K., Bourgon, G., Helmus, L., & Hodgson, S. (2009). The principles of effective correctional treatment also apply to sexual offenders: A meta-analysis. *Criminal Justice and Behavior, 36*(9), 865–891.

Harkins, L., Flak, V. E., Beech, A. R., & Woodhams, J. (2012). Evaluation of a community-based sex offender treatment program using a good lives model approach. *Sexual Abuse*, 24(6), 519–543.

Henwood, K. S., Chou, S., & Browne, K. D. (2015). A systematic review and meta-analysis on the effectiveness of CBT informed anger management. *Aggression and Violent Behavior*, 25, 280–292.

Her Majesty's Inspectorate of Probation. (2017). *An inspection of through the gate resettlement services for prisoners serving 12 months or more.* https://www.justiceinspectorates.gov.uk/cjji/inspections/throughthegate2/

Heynen, E., Hoogsteder, L., Van Vugt, E., Schalkwijk, F., Stams, G. J., & Assink, M. (2023). Effectiveness of moral developmental interventions for youth engaged in delinquent behavior: A meta-analysis. *International Journal of Offender Therapy and Comparative Criminology*. https://doi.org/10.1177/0306624X231172648

Hollin, C. R., & Palmer, E. J. (2009). Cognitive skills programmes for offenders. *Psychology, Crime and Law*, 15(2–3), 147–164.

Kosson, D. S., Walsh, Z., Anderson, J. R., Brook, M., Swogger, M. T., & Verborg, R. (2019). Evaluation of a cognitive-behavioral intervention for high- and medium-risk probationers. *Behavioral Sciences & the Law*, 37(4), 329–341.

Lipsey, M. W., Landenberger, N. A., & Wilson, S. J. (2007). *Effects of cognitive-behavioral programs for criminal offenders.* The Cambell Collaboration.

Little, G. L., & Robinson, K. D. (1988). Moral reconation therapy: A systematic step-by-step treatment system for treatment resistant clients. *Psychological Reports*, 62(1), 135–151.

Lutz, M., Zani, D., Fritz, M., Dudeck, M., & Franke, I. (2022). A review and comparative analysis of the risk-needs-responsivity, good lives, and recovery models in forensic psychiatric treatment. *Frontiers in Psychiatry*, 13, 988905.

Martinson, R. (1974). What works? Questions and answers about prison reform. *Public Interest*, 35(2), 22–54.

Maruna, S. (2001). *Making good* (Vol. 86). American Psychological Association.

Morse, S. J., Wright, K. A., & Klapow, M. (2022). Correctional rehabilitation and positive psychology: Opportunities and challenges. *Sociology Compass*, 16(3), e12960.

Ogloff, J. R., & Davis, M. R. (2004). Advances in offender assessment and rehabilitation: Contributions of the risk–needs–responsivity approach. *Psychology, Crime and Law, 10*(3), 229–242.

Polaschek, D. L. (2012). An appraisal of the risk–need–responsivity (RNR) model of offender rehabilitation and its application in correctional treatment. *Legal and Criminological Psychology, 17*(1), 1–17.

Prescott, D. S., & Willis, G. M. (2022). Using the good lives model (GLM) in clinical practice: Lessons learned from international implementation projects. *Aggression and Violent Behavior, 63*, 101717.

Ribeiro da Silva, D., Rijo, D., Salekin, R. T., Paulo, M., Miguel, R., & Gilbert, P. (2021). Clinical change in psychopathic traits after the PSYCHOPATHY. COMP program: Preliminary findings of a controlled trial with male detained youth. *Journal of Experimental Criminology, 17*, 397–421.

Sampson, R. J., & Laub, J. H. (2003). Desistance from crime over the life course. In J. T. Mortimer & M. J. Shanahan (Eds.), *Handbook of the life course, Handbooks of sociology and social research* (pp. 295–309). Springer. https://doi.org/10.1007/978-0-306-48247-2_14

Seewald, K., Rossegger, A., Gerth, J., Urbaniok, F., Phillips, G., & Endrass, J. (2018). Effectiveness of a risk–need–responsivity-based treatment program for violent and sexual offenders: Results of a retrospective, quasi-experimental study. *Legal and Criminological Psychology, 23*(1), 85–99.

Taylor, J., Akerman, G., & Hocken, K. (2020). Cultivating compassion focussed practice for those who have committed sexual offences. *Sexual Crime and Trauma*, 57–83.

Taylor, J., & Hocken, K. (2021). Hurt people hurt people: Using a trauma sensitive and compassion focused approach to support people to understand and manage their criminogenic needs. *Journal of Forensic Practice, 23*(3), 301–315.

Taylor, J., & Hocken, K. (2024). Illuminating the dark side: Life story and formulation work to understand criminogenic capacities and human harmfulness. *Abuse: An International Impact Journal, 5*(1), 46–60.

Viglione, J. (2019). The risk-need-responsivity model: How do probation officers implement the principles of effective intervention? *Criminal Justice and Behavior, 46*(5), 655–673.

Vojt, G., Thomson, L. D. G., & Marshall, L. A. (2013). The predictive validity of the HCR-20 following clinical implementation: Does it work in practice? *Journal of Forensic Psychiatry and Psychology*, 24(3), 371–385. https://doi.org/10.1080/14789949.2013.800894

Ward, T., Arrigo, B., Barnao, M., Beech, A., Brown, D. A., Cording, J., Day, A., Durrant, R., Gannon, T. A., Hart, S. D., Prescott, D., Strauss-Hughes, A., Tamatea, A., & Taxman, F. (2022). Urgent issues and prospects in correctional rehabilitation practice and research. *Legal and Criminological Psychology*, 27(2), 103–128. https://doi.org/10.1111/lcrp.12211

Ward, T., & Gannon, T. A. (2006). Rehabilitation, etiology, and self-regulation: The comprehensive good lives model of treatment for sexual offenders. *Aggression and Violent Behavior*, 11(1), 77–94.

Ward, T., & Maruna, S. (2007). *Key ideas in criminology. Rehabilitation: Beyond the risk paradigm*. Routledge.

Ward, T., Yates, P. M., & Willis, G. M. (2012). The good lives model and the risk need responsivity model: A critical response to Andrews, Bonta, and Wormith (2011). *Criminal Justice and Behavior*, 39(1), 94–110.

Webster, C. D., Douglas, K. S., Eaves, D., & Hart, S. D. (1997). *HCR-20: Assessing risk for violence, version 2*. Mental Health, Law, and Policy Institute, Simon Fraser University.

Willis, G. M., Prescott, D. S., & Yates, P. M. (2013). The good lives model (GLM) in theory and practice. *Sexual Abuse in Australia and New Zealand*, 5(1), 3–9.

Willis, G., & Ward, T. (2013). The good lives model: Evidence that it works. In L. Craig, L. Dixon, & T. A. Gannon (Eds.), *What works in offender rehabilitation: An evidence-based approach to assessment and treatment* (pp. 305–318). John Wiley & Son.

Yates, P. M. (2013). Treatment of sexual offenders: Research, best practices, and emerging models. *International Journal of Behavioral Consultation and Therapy*, 8(3–4), 89.

Zeccola, J., Kelty, S. F., & Boer, D. (2021). Does the good lives model work? A systematic review of the recidivism evidence. *Journal of Forensic Practice*, 23(3), 285–300.

4

COMPASSION-FOCUSED THERAPY/ COMPASSIONATE MIND TRAINING THEORY

ABSTRACT

This chapter delves into the 'East' of the theoretical and practical background of the COMPASS model, particularly in relation to compassion. It specifically examines Compassion-Focused Therapy (CFT) as a therapeutic method for working with individuals who have offended, explaining how offending behaviour develops and how it can be managed. This is achieved through tried-and-tested techniques for cultivating a compassionate mind. The information presented here provides the theoretical foundations for the compassion component of the model.

Keywords: Compassion; compassionate mind; Compassion-Focused Therapy; emotional regulation; self-compassion

UNDERSTANDING THE DARK SIDE OF THE MIND IN RELATION TO OFFENDING BEHAVIOUR

We all have the potential for kindness and compassion, yet we also harbour a darker side of the mind that can lead us to actions society deems bad or wrong. Like the old Native America Indian tale of the two wolves, it depends on which one you feed. This dark side can torment us and shape our feelings into behaviours that harm ourselves or others, turning retaliation into torture, anger into assault or rage into murder (Gilbert, 2018). Compassion-Focused Therapy (CFT) recognises that our minds evolved or depending on your beliefs were created with ancestral survival mindsets that shape our present behaviour. Beneath our newly developed brains lies the old brain, evolved to help us survive by any means necessary. We all want to flourish and see those around us thrive. Simultaneously, we seek to acquire resources to overcome threats to our existence. We are hardwired to protect what is ours, including the people around us and our possessions, both external (property, family) and internal (pride, respect). Our minds are equipped with a set of needs, wants, desires, preferences and goals that our environments can influence for good or ill.

Social dominance can make us ruthless in our pursuit of competitiveness and superiority. When viewed this way, offending behaviour can be seen as a method to acquire resources for survival, improve social ranking and avoid feelings of inferiority and shame. History shows that while humans are capable of great achievements, they are responsible for some of the most horrendous actions on earth. Delving into the dark recesses of our minds and taking responsibility for our actions is a true act of courage, which is why compassion is a great motivator for change. It is important for those working with offenders to move away from the dichotomy of good and bad people and recognise that everyone has a dark side. From a CFT perspective, the goal is to understand why someone acts from their dark side instead of their more compassionate, caring and cooperative side (Ribeiro da Silva & Rijo, 2022).

Compassion in criminal and forensic settings is controversial because it asks that people who have committed offences be treated kindly. Some members of the public argue that offenders deserve only punishment, not compassion. This sentiment is echoed in the political sphere, where certain groups believe the best way to reduce offending is to incarcerate criminals. This approach benefits governments and political parties during elections. The victims of crimes and their families, affected by drugs, violence, rape and murder, understandably want harsh punishment. However, re-offending rates continue to increase with this punitive approach to crime. A positive, compassionate approach is hoped to provide a different, potentially more long-term, and effective solution to reducing and perhaps even stopping offending in our society.

THE ORIGINS OF CFT AND COMPASSIONATE MIND TRAINING (CMT)

CFT was developed by Professor Paul Gilbert, a clinical psychologist in the United Kingdom who worked with individuals experiencing high levels of shame and guilt (Gilbert, 2009). CFT combines Buddhist principles of compassion with evidence-based research in attachment theory, social psychology, neuroscience, evolution and developmental psychology. It has been shown to be effective for a range of mental and physical conditions, helping people flourish and improve their well-being (Kirby, 2017). CFT operates on the premise that individuals can build resilience to shame by enhancing their ability to self-soothe and practice compassion. Unlike Cognitive Behavioural Therapy (CBT), CFT facilitates a compassionate understanding of past offending motivations and encourages the acknowledgement of remorse and guilt. It is grounded in three key theoretical ideas about the evolution of our brains and the impact of emotions on behaviour.

KEY THEORETICAL IDEAS IN CFT

There are three key ideas of CFT in relation to offending and anti-social behaviour. These ideas are tricky brains, self-identity shaped by genes and sociocultural experiences and an emotional regulation system that significantly impacts offending behaviour.

Tricky Brains

According to CFT, our brains have evolved with both primitive (old brains) and complex (new brains) capabilities. The old brain, associated with the limbic system, is a product of millions of years of evolution (or creation, depending on beliefs) and shares motivations with other primates, such as nurturing, seeking food, sex, status, attachment and protection (survival). This brain is responsible for basic emotions like anger, sadness, anxiety, disgust and joy.

Over the last two million years, humans evolved a set of new, intelligent cognitive capabilities, creating more complex and sophisticated thinking abilities. These include imagination, reasoning and self-monitoring, which allow us to reflect on the past, anticipate the future and form beliefs about our thoughts, feelings and behaviour. This can shape our sense of identity and how we see ourselves in the world. Despite these advancements, our old and new brains can get caught in unhelpful 'Mind Loops', causing difficulties and making us vulnerable to criminogenic needs. Teaching clients about these mind loops and asking them to explain their experiences can help them understand their thought patterns, especially in the context of offending.

Self-identity Shaped by Genes and Sociocultural Experiences

Interaction between genes and environment: CFT/CMT helps individuals understand that self-identity results from the interaction between genes and social circumstances. Different experiences shape brain development, and environments can affect gene expression, biology and physiology. Offenders often have negative self-identities, believing they were 'born bad' or are irredeemable 'junkies'. This can become a self-fulfilling prophecy. It's crucial to remember that we don't choose our genes or our early environments, and we often don't choose our experiences. Our current self is just one version of many possible selves.

An example of how this can be used with someone who is desisting is to ask them to imagine how they would have been if they had grown up in a loving, caring and supportive environment with lots of growth opportunities. Imagine that they had been raised by parents who gave them lots of attention, support and encouragement, and they got whatever they wanted without having to turn to offending to get it. They can be invited to imagine the feelings (warmth, care, compassion, security) and behaviour they would be experiencing and the relationships they would have (supportive, positive, caring and helpful). Even though we don't know for sure that they would be different, they may be very likely not to be addicted to drugs or have issues with anger and deviancy. They would most likely be driven towards pro-social behaviours rather than offending because they have all their basic needs met. If we create different experiences, then another version of us will emerge into the world. This helps us recognise that our experiences were shaped for us and not by us. While it can be easy to blame ourselves or what has happened to us for our behaviour, we can change who we are now and take responsibility for the things we have been through and make positive changes to our lives. CFT can involve exercises where offenders imagine growing up in a loving, supportive environment and how different they would be. This can help them realise that their experiences shaped their current behaviour, and that they have the power to change their future.

Emotional Regulation Systems

CFT simplifies the complex functional emotions into three major systems: threat, drive and soothing.

Threat and self-protection system: This system alerts us to threats and helps us respond appropriately, involving emotions like anger, anxiety and disgust.

It is designed to protect us from harm. Offenders often see the world as hostile, believing their criminal behaviours are necessary for survival.

Drive/Seeking System: This system stimulates desires and directs goals to acquire essential resources for survival, such as food, sex, friendships and shelter. It is associated with joy and motivates us to seek things that bring pleasure and help us flourish. When balanced with compassion, it focuses attention on pro-social goals.

Soothing/Contentment System: This system allows us to rest and relax, enjoy low-energy activities and feel safe. It's responsible for balancing the other two systems and is sensitive to care and compassion from others. A poorly functioning soothing system can lead individuals to unhealthy external sources like substances or alcohol to self-soothe. CFT aims to develop healthy self-soothing techniques and increase self-compassion.

THE INTERACTION BETWEEN DRIVE AND THREAT SYSTEMS IN RELATION TO OFFENDING BEHAVIOUR

The threat and drive systems can interact, motivating individuals towards negative goals. For example, someone might seek material possessions or social status to avoid feeling inferior or safe. They might use manipulation to gain approval or feel superior. In Western societies, there's a focus on self-gain and material needs, leading to behaviours like theft, drug dealing and gang affiliation. Offenders might compete for status within gangs or use manipulation and violence to alleviate feelings of inferiority or demonstrate power. This behaviour often stems from a threat-based drive, where violence becomes a means of survival and social status. However, these actions are driven by a need to escape feelings of anxiety, stress and depression. Understanding the threat-based drive helps us see why someone engages in offending behaviour and highlights where compassion is needed to alleviate distress and support desistance.

PRACTICAL APPLICATION: THE THREE CIRCLES

The three circles can be used as an informal method to understand our emotional lives and actions. This method involves drawing out the emotional regulation systems with coloured pens to represent their intensity. It can be used to examine present emotions, past influences and future goals.

Formulating these systems helps individuals recognise how their experiences shape their actions and helps guide them towards healthier emotional regulation. By understanding and balancing these three systems, CFT aims to help individuals develop a compassionate mind, which can lead to more pro-social behaviours and reduce offending.

COMPASSION-FOCUSED FORMULATION

A more formal four-column formulation can be used to help make sense of past threat-drive experiences. This approach involves examining:

Key Life Experiences

These are significant events or circumstances from an individual's past that have shaped their psychological and emotional landscape. These might include experiences of poverty, abuse, neglect, Adverse Childhood Experiences (ACES) or other forms of trauma.

Development of Threats and Fears

Key life experiences can lead to the development of specific threats and fears. For instance, growing up in poverty might create a fear of scarcity and a sense of shame and low social ranking.

Safety Strategies

To manage these threats and fears, individuals develop safety strategies. These strategies are behaviours or thought patterns intended to protect oneself from perceived dangers. In the context of offending behaviour, a safety strategy might be engaging in criminal activities like selling drugs or committing theft to obtain wealth and elevate social status.

Unintended Consequences

While these safety strategies might temporarily mitigate threats and fears, they often lead to unintended consequences. For example, offending behaviour might result in being labelled as an offender, leading to stigma and internal conflict between the self and the perceived social self. Additionally, being caught and convicted leads to a criminal record, creating further barriers to desistance and reintegration into society.

EXAMPLE APPLICATION

Consider an individual who grew up in poverty. This key life experience might lead to feelings of shame and a perceived lower social ranking (threats and fears). To manage these feelings, the individual might resort to selling drugs or robbing others (safety strategies) to gain wealth and social status. However, these actions result in unintended consequences: being labelled an offender, experiencing stigma and ultimately receiving a criminal record, which further hinders their ability to desist from crime and reintegrate into society. By using this four-column formulation, therapists and individuals can better understand how past experiences contribute to current behaviours and develop more effective, compassionate strategies for change. This perspective helps to reframe offending behaviour as a by-product of attempts to cope with historical threats and fears, encouraging a more compassionate and constructive approach to rehabilitation.

OVERCOMING FEARS, BLOCKS AND RESISTANCE TO COMPASSION

When working with individuals who have offended, their harsh upbringing and traumatic experiences often lead to fears, blocks and resistance to compassion (Gilbert, 2017; Ribeiro da Silva et al., 2015). Exploring their past, present and future can evoke difficult emotions, such as:

- *Anxiety and fear*: Individuals may worry about their future and whether they can truly change.

- *Sadness*: Reflecting on past experiences and actions can bring about deep sadness.

- *Guilt, remorse and shame*: These emotions often arise when individuals look back at their lives and acknowledge the harm they've caused and endured.

COMMON BARRIERS TO COMPASSION

- *Reluctance to Change:* The journey towards change involves confronting painful truths and overcoming significant obstacles, such as the fear of failing to desist from offending or facing stigma and ridicule from others.

- *Belief of Undeserved Compassion:* Many individuals believe they don't deserve compassion because of their actions or lack of compassionate experiences in life. As a consequence of the threat-drive mind, people who offend can get stuck in a cycle of blame and shame, believing they are a bad person because of their offences and deserve to be punished for their actions. Negative self-criticism can lead to a lack of responsibility for what they have done and prevent them from considering themselves worthy of compassion. However, it is during or after our struggles that the strength of compassion can help us accept our difficult feelings, understand our negative experiences, grow from them and find a way out of our suffering.

- *Perception of Compassion as Weakness:* There is a common misconception that being compassionate and kind to oneself is a sign of weakness, making one vulnerable to exploitation. When working on ourselves and developing compassion, it takes a lot of mental courage to build the emotional and physical strength we need to manage the pains of the past and the fears that come from making positive changes in our lives. Compassion helps us tolerate the discomfort of painful memories, the difficulties of leaving parts of our lives behind and the anxiety we have about the future. It makes us resilient and wise as we navigate the desistance journey.

- *Compassion gets me off the hook for what I have done:* It can be easy to think that a compassionate approach to offending behaviour would involve people being let off or forgiven for what they have done without having to take responsibility. However, as we have discussed, this is not the case. In fact, developing a compassionate mind means doing the opposite. It gives people the skills to accept what they have done and to take responsibility for their offending behaviour, manage the distress of being open and honest with themselves and find a way forward on their desistance journey.

STRATEGIES TO OVERCOME RESISTANCE

Embody compassionate understanding: Practitioners must demonstrate a compassionate understanding of their client's feelings and experiences, validating them without judgement. This helps create a safe space for clients to explore their emotions.

Use skills and attributes of a compassionate mind: Practitioners should model and teach the skills of a compassionate mind, including empathy, mindfulness and self-compassion.

Explore past experiences with courageous compassion: Understanding how past experiences have shaped present feelings of shame and anger can be transformative. This involves:

Recognising unintended consequences: Helping individuals see that their current feelings and behaviours are often unintended consequences of factors beyond their control.

Reframing experiences: Encouraging a compassionate reframing of their experiences, emphasising that they can change and overcome their fears and resistance with compassion skills.

WHAT IS COMPASSION?

What is compassion anyway, and where does this word we hear so often come from? Compassion derives from two Latin 'Compati', which translates as 'to be with suffering'. While compassion requires that we be with someone's suffering, or our own, simply being with it does not always help rid us or others of suffering. Considering this inaccuracy the definition of compassion has been adapted to include the awareness and motivation to act upon suffering. Therefore, one of the most common and universally accepted definitions of compassion is a 'sensitivity to suffering in self and others, with a commitment to alleviate and prevent it' (Gilbert, 2014, p. 19). Compassion in this conceptualisation has two psychologies, one is an awareness of suffering and the other the motivation to do something about it. To do this, the attributes, strengths and skills of compassion must be developed.

ATTRIBUTES OF COMPASSION

The first psychology contains a set of attributes that help us notice suffering and engage in distress.

- Care for well-being and our motivation to care about ourselves and others.

- Sensitivity is our ability to notice and become more open to suffering and be moved towards it rather than ignoring or avoiding it.

- Sympathy involves being emotionally moved by our own and another's pain and suffering.

- To do this effectively, we need to be able to tolerate distress (distress tolerance) and the painful memories that remind us of our difficult experiences.

- Empathy allows us to tune into these feelings and make sense of them. This helps us take a deeper look at where our suffering comes from and better understand it.

- Finally, because our 'tricky brains' cause us to behave in certain ways that we or others find difficult to understand, we want to adopt a compassionate non-judgement towards our and others' behaviour. This enables us to accept things without criticising or condoning what we or others have done, no matter how cruel or harmful. Even if we want to change, this approach can give us perspective and the motivation to do things differently by not judging the complex minds that we have.

THE SKILLS AND STRENGTHS OF COMPASSION THAT CAN HELP WITH DESISTANCE

The second psychology focuses on the skills and wisdom needed to develop the attributes of a compassionate mind. These skills can be used when working with the difficult life experiences of people who have offended and helping them imagine a different future. This is about developing the courage, wisdom and strength for helpful self and other compassionate behaviour rather than harmful offending behaviour. It is important to consider the difficulties with this for people who have experienced abusive or traumatic backgrounds. When supporting people who have offended towards developing compassion, it is important to remind them that our behaviour is not always our fault but a result of genes, upbringing and sociocultural factors. Using examples of what compassion is, and the courage it takes to be compassionate, and the benefits it has for increasing our well-being are crucial for developing this understanding. This can help them develop the courage to take responsibility for their actions and to live in a way that is more pro-social. One of the reasons for this block to the flow of compassion (to self, others and from others) are feelings of shame that come from unresolved traumas and pain from past experiences. This can prevent them from being compassionate to others for the pain they caused, to themselves for the pain they feel and from others to help with their suffering (Ribeiro da Silva et al., 2019).

PREPARING THE MIND FOR COMPASSION

Although we may not believe we can change our minds, evidence suggests that our brains are more malleable than was previously thought (Gilbert, 2009). Through mindful attention and soothing rhythm breathing exercises, we can adapt our thinking and what we pay attention to and start to activate the soothing system. If the focus is always on the threat or threat-drive system, the person is more likely to feel anxious, fearful and aggressive. In reducing this and reducing the threat system, the goal of compassion is to stimulate the soothing system and strengthen the impact it has on them. Like all muscles in the body, developing a compassionate mind takes practice. This does not have to be much to begin with, but a little each day is a good starting point. It is helpful to start the process from a place of comfort where we feel grounded.

Compassionate Attention

Compassionate attention involves shifting our attention in a way that is more helpful to us. An example could be remembering when we have shown compassion to others, or when someone has been kind to us. This can be a good way to reassure someone who has a history of criminality that they are not a bad person, or if a person has experienced abuse from others, that not everyone has malicious intentions or is out to get them. It can be used to help identify their positive attributes and remind them of their strengths such as resilience and courage towards setbacks, as well as relieve them of a dominant threat system.

Compassionate Reasoning

We all experience different mindsets from time to time, which take us through a range of emotions. For example, if we are angry, we might only pay attention to what or who made us angry. Our thoughts become focused on that thing or person, and we ruminate about revenge or fantasise about what we will do to them. We may even hit out if we have the chance. Later, we might regret this and feel uncomfortable with our actions, all the while beating ourselves up for what we did, ruminating on getting caught and what will happen if we do. Compassionate reasoning refers to the ways in which we think about ourselves, the world and others. Reasoning skills allow us to consider alternative viewpoints and ways of looking at things. Compassionate reasoning encourages us to do this with kind, helpful and supportive thoughts. Mood states play a big part in our reasoning and how we reflect on our current and future selves. Despite their negative associations, shame and self-critical thinking can be considered helpful to some and difficult to change. Compassionate reasoning is therefore encouraged as a helpful alternative to self-critical self-talk. This can be used to make sense of the reasons why someone has offended, and while it is not their fault, it is their responsibility to change.

Compassionate Behaviour

Compassionate behaviour involves acting in ways that advance our life's journey, reduce suffering for ourselves and others and foster personal growth and flourishing. It can be directed both towards oneself and others. Behaving compassionately encompasses treating oneself with kindness and understanding. This means being gentle with oneself during times of difficulty or failure and acknowledging one's own needs for care and support. For example, showing self-compassion might involve engaging in self-care practices, forgiving oneself for past mistakes and setting healthy boundaries. Compassionate behaviour also includes having the courage to make challenging decisions that may not offer immediate rewards but are essential for long-term well-being. This could mean resisting pressure from friends to participate in harmful activities, such as gang fights or theft when you are striving to make positive changes in your life. It involves assertiveness, standing up for oneself and others respectfully and clearly and making choices that align with one's values and goals. While avoidance might seem like a helpful response by providing temporary relief, it is often short-lived and does not address the underlying issues. Compassionate behaviour involves confronting challenges directly and making decisions that support personal growth and well-being. In everyday life, compassionate behaviour can manifest as offering support to a friend in need, standing up against injustice and helping those who are suffering. Integrating compassion into daily interactions helps build resilience, enhance relationships and contribute positively to one's own development and that of others.

Compassionate Imagery

Our brains can imagine something and stimulate feelings in us. For example, we can imagine something bad is going to happen and feel anxious. We can also have fantasies about someone we are attracted to, and those thoughts will create a physiological effect on our bodies. To use compassionate imagery means to imagine what a compassionate person would look like, how they would behave, the thoughts they would have, what they would feel, what they would sound like and the tone of voice they would use. What comes to mind can be imagined with warmth, non-judgement, strength and wisdom. Engaging in these exercises and daily practice imagining the self as a compassionate person can help generate compassionate feelings for the self. Our brains can imagine something and stimulate feelings in us. The goal is to create an image of an ideal compassionate self and a pro-social self-identity and imagine what we would be doing and how we would behave until we make it happen in reality.

Compassionate Feeling

Compassionate feelings refer to our ability to generate compassion feelings for ourselves, for others and from others. They can help us tolerate suffering, improve our well-being and help us flourish. We can generate feelings of contentment, kindness, warmth, by wishing that we and others are free of suffering and can live a happy life. Wishing the best for others who have harmed us is associated with forgiveness, and it can be liberating, in the same way wishing ourselves compassion for past transgressions can free us of the same and guilt of our offender pasts. This is achieved through directing compassion to the self as well as others.

Compassionate Sensation

Compassionate sensation refers to the way in which we can consider using all our senses, such as touch, smell and hearing, to stimulate positive emotions and compassion. When we focus on our bodily senses in ways that engage our soothing system, we can regulate our distress. For example, breathing exercises can help the body slow down. Also, adopting certain body postures can activate physical states to help us feel stronger, balanced and more grounded. This can be helpful when getting to grips with a new non-offender identity and working to change the parts of the self that are associated with past offending behaviour.

FLOW OF COMPASSION

There are three flows of compassion that can be helpful with developing a compassionate mind. This involves imaging compassion flowing, inwardly from others, outwardly to others and probably the most difficult of all, from the self to the self, or self-compassion.

Compassion Flowing In

Compassion flowing into you from others requires that we accept compassion from others and allow that to help with increasing the soothing system. Linking this to the past, we can imagine times when someone showed compassion to us and how that made us feel.

Compassion Flowing Out

Compassion flowing out to others is how we direct our compassion to those around us. This can be family, friends, the community or even the whole world. We can do this by our behaviours and the way we communicate to others or by wanting or wishing that others be happy and free from suffering.

Compassion Flowing to the Self

Self-compassion is probably the most difficult of the three flows as it involves directing compassion to the self. Kirsten Neff (2003) suggests that when having doubts about self-compassion, we think about a friend who is struggling like we are and what we would say to them. In most cases, we would be supportive and use encouraging language towards them. The idea is to then take this support and direct it to self and treat ourselves as we would a friend. After all, no one is closer to us than ourselves. The good thing is we can learn how to direct more compassion to ourselves and develop the skills of self-compassion.

CONCLUSION

Preventing a return to offending is the primary goal of any intervention aimed at individuals who have offended. In CFT and the COMPASS model, this focus is on cultivating the skills of compassion to overcome barriers and setbacks on the path to desistance from offending. The aim of a compassion-focused intervention is to help individuals understand that suffering and distress are inherent parts of life. There will always be obstacles that can hinder progress, but the key is to do our best despite these challenges. Compassionate interventions emphasise that everyone makes mistakes, and that perfection is unattainable. We are all fallible human beings navigating a complex world with limited understanding of our own minds. Expecting ourselves to navigate life without errors or setbacks is unrealistic and sets us up for failure. Accepting our own flaws and those of others helps us appreciate our shared humanity. Developing a compassionate mindset, supported by compassionate practitioners, is crucial for finding a path away from offending and towards desistance. While life may have presented us with challenges and shaped our experiences, we are responsible for making amends for our actions and the harm we have caused to others and ourselves. Embracing our imperfections and learning to approach life with compassion can guide us towards a more positive and fulfilling future.

REFERENCES

Gilbert, P. (2009). Introducing compassion-focused therapy. *Advances in Psychiatric Treatment, 15*(3), 199–208.

Gilbert, P. (2014). The origins and nature of compassion focused therapy. *British Journal of Clinical Psychology, 53*(1), 6–41.

Gilbert, P. (2017). Exploring compassion focused therapy in forensic settings: An evolutionary and social-contextual approach. In J. Davies & C. Nagi (Eds.), *Individual psychological therapies in forensic settings: Research and practice* (pp. 59–84). Routledge/Taylor & Francis Group. https://doi.org/10.4324/9781315666136-5

Gilbert, P. (2018). Forward. In R. L. Kolts, T. Bell, J. Bennett-Levy, & C. Irons (Eds.), *Experiencing compassion-focused therapy from the inside out: A self-practice/self-reflection workbook for therapists* (pp. vii–xvi). Guilford Publications.

Kirby, J. N. (2017). Compassion interventions: The programmes, the evidence, and implications for research and practice. *Psychology and Psychotherapy: Theory, Research and Practice, 90*(3), 432–455.

Neff, K. D. (2003). Self-compassion: An alternative conceptualization of a healthy attitude toward oneself. *Self and Identity, 2*(2), 85–101. https://doi.org/10.1080/15298860309032

Ribeiro da Silva, D., & Rijo, D. (2022). Compassion focused therapy in forensic settings. In P. Gilbert & G. Simos (Eds.), *Compassion focused therapy: Clinical practice and applications* (pp. 505–518). Routledge.

Ribeiro da Silva, D., Rijo, D., Castilho, P., & Gilbert, P. (2019). The efficacy of a compassion-focused therapy–based intervention in reducing psychopathic traits and disruptive behavior: A clinical case study with a juvenile detainee. *Clinical Case Studies, 18*(5), 323–343.

Ribeiro da Silva, D., Rijo, D., & Salekin, R. T. (2015). The evolutionary roots of psychopathy. *Aggression and Violent Behavior, 21*, 85–96.

5

POSITIVE PSYCHOLOGY THEORY AND PRACTICE

ABSTRACT

This chapter examines the 'West' of the Compassionate Positive Applied Strengths-based Solutions (COMPASS) model and application of Positive Psychology to understanding and supporting desistance from offending behaviour. Positive Psychology, a field dedicated to the study of strengths, well-being and human flourishing, offers valuable tools for fostering pro-social change in individuals with a history of offending. Unlike positive criminality, which focuses on rehabilitative strategies within the criminal justice system, Positive Psychology emphasises enhancing overall life satisfaction through the cultivation of personal strengths and positive experiences. This chapter discusses the concept of well-being, the Positive Emotions, Engagement, Relationships, Meaning and Accomplishment (PERMA) model and the Broaden and Build theory, highlighting their relevance to desistance. It also explores key skills and strengths, such as hope, character strengths and gratitude, that can support individuals in their journey towards a life free from offending. By integrating these principles, this chapter provides a framework for understanding how personal growth and positive psychological attributes can contribute to successful desistance and improved quality of life.

Keywords: Strengths; hope; optimism; flourishing; authentic happiness; PERMA

POSITIVE PSYCHOLOGY: ORIGINS AND DEFINITION

Positive Psychology is a branch of psychology focused on understanding and promoting what makes life meaningful and fulfilling. Unlike traditional psychology, which often concentrates on pathology and what goes wrong, Positive Psychology explores strengths, well-being and human flourishing. It is concerned with fostering positive emotions, character strengths and a sense of purpose. Defined as 'the scientific study of what makes life most worth living' (Peterson, 2008), Positive Psychology was first introduced by Abraham Maslow (1954) and further developed by Martin Seligman. Seligman's (2019) approach was a response to the narrow focus of clinical psychology on mental illness, aiming instead to highlight what is right with people and how they can flourish. This approach is crucial for individuals with offending behaviour, as it helps shift focus from past mistakes to personal growth and positive development, facilitating rehabilitation and reintegration into society.

DISTINCTION FROM POSITIVE CRIMINOLOGY

While Positive Psychology and positive criminology share common goals, they differ in scope and application. Positive criminology, a term introduced by Ronel (2015), adapts Positive Psychology principles to address criminal behaviour specifically. It integrates theories from psychology, criminology, sociology and criminal justice to promote positive change in offenders by emphasising their strengths and potential for reform. Positive criminology targets specific at-risk groups, aiming to balance traditional criminological views with an understanding of offenders' potential for positive change. In contrast, Positive Psychology applies more broadly, focusing on general well-being and strengths applicable to all individuals, including those with offending histories. Both fields aim to improve life satisfaction and prevent crime but approach these goals from different angles.

SCIENTIFIC UNDERSTANDING OF WELL-BEING AND ITS RELEVANCE TO OFFENDING BEHAVIOUR

Positive Psychology identifies key factors contributing to well-being, which are essential for all individuals, including those with offending behaviour.

Well-being encompasses aspects of life that lead to positive feelings and satisfaction. It is generally categorised into two types: hedonic and eudemonic.

Hedonic well-being: This aspect focuses on pleasure and avoidance of pain, reflecting a subjective experience of positive and negative emotions. Hedonic well-being, or subjective well-being, involves high positive affect, low negative affect and overall life satisfaction. While seeking pleasure can enhance well-being, it can sometimes lead to negative consequences, such as addiction or health issues, as seen with drug use.

Eudemonic well-being: In contrast, eudemonic well-being centres on finding purpose and meaning in life. Originating from ancient Greek philosophy, it is about reaching one's true potential and achieving a sense of fulfilment. For individuals with offending behaviour, discovering a sense of purpose can be transformative, helping them move beyond past actions and find new, constructive paths.

Positive Psychology provides a framework for understanding and fostering well-being through strengths and positive emotions, which is particularly relevant for those seeking to overcome offending behaviour. By focusing on personal growth and life satisfaction, Positive Psychology can support desistance and reintegration, complementing the goals of positive criminology and contributing to more effective rehabilitation and societal reintegration.

AUTHENTIC HAPPINESS AND ITS RELEVANCE TO OFFENDING BEHAVIOUR

In his seminal work, Authentic Happiness (2002), Martin Seligman identifies three distinct paths to achieving happiness:

The pleasant life: This path, aligned with hedonic well-being, focuses on maximising pleasurable experiences. It emphasises the development of skills that enhance positive emotions and minimise discomfort. Although seeking pleasure is a component of happiness, it is only one aspect of a fulfilling life.

The Good Life: Centred on the use of personal strengths in activities that bring satisfaction and enrichment, this path is associated with experiencing 'flow', a state of deep engagement and absorption in an activity (Csikszentmihalyi, 2002). Engaging in activities that align with one's authentic strengths contributes to overall life satisfaction.

The meaningful life: This path involves pursuing goals that contribute to something greater than oneself, such as using personal strengths for the benefit of others. It reflects a sense of purpose and connection to a broader context.

When combined with the Good Life, it aligns with eudemonic well-being, where life satisfaction is derived from living with purpose and contributing to the welfare of others.

For individuals with offending behaviour, considering all three paths to happiness is crucial. While pursuing a Good Life is valuable, integrating elements of Pleasant and Meaningful Lives can enhance personal fulfilment and foster a sense of human connection beyond self-interest.

THE POSITIVE EMOTIONS, ENGAGEMENT, RELATIONSHIPS, MEANING AND ACCOMPLISHMENT (PERMA) MODEL

Martin Seligman's later development of the authentic happiness model into the PERMA model (2011) outlines five key elements that contribute to well-being:

Positive Emotions: Experiencing positive emotions like happiness is linked to decreased criminal behaviour. High life satisfaction is associated with a lower likelihood of engaging in crime, while low satisfaction can correlate with higher crime rates (Olson et al., 2021). Understanding how to cultivate lasting happiness through pro-social means is essential for preventing re-offending.

Engagement: This refers to being fully immersed in activities that bring joy and fulfilment. Engagement is related to experiencing flow and can involve work, education or positive leisure activities. Participation in meaningful and enjoyable activities, especially within social groups, enhances well-being and can help steer individuals away from offending behaviour.

Relationships (Positive/Pro-social): Building and maintaining positive relationships is fundamental to well-being. Strong social connections contribute to happiness and a sense of belonging. For individuals re-entering society, developing compassionate and supportive relationships can facilitate successful reintegration and reduce the likelihood of re-offending (McNeill & Schinkel, 2024).

Meaning: Finding a sense of purpose and contributing to something greater than oneself provides a deeper sense of fulfilment. It involves aligning personal values with life goals and reflecting on one's role in the broader community. Meaningful pursuits can help individuals with offending behaviour develop a pro-social identity and find motivation for positive change (Maruna, 2001).

Accomplishments/Achievements: Achieving goals and experiencing a sense of pride and fulfilment from accomplishments are key to authentic happiness. Setting and reaching desistance goals can enhance overall well-being and foster a sense of achievement. The PERMA model suggests that focusing on these five elements can lead to flourishing and improved life satisfaction.

Applying the principles of authentic happiness and the PERMA model to individuals with offending behaviour can offer valuable insights and rehabilitation strategies. By addressing pleasure, engagement, relationships, meaning and accomplishments, offenders can work towards a more fulfilling and pro-social life, thereby supporting their journey towards desistance and reintegration into society.

SELF-DETERMINATION THEORY (SDT) AND ITS RELEVANCE FOR OFFENDING BEHAVIOUR

SDT, developed by Ryan and Deci (2000), provides a comprehensive framework for understanding human motivation by emphasising three core psychological needs: autonomy, competence and relatedness. According to SDT, satisfying these needs fosters positive motivation, personal growth and overall well-being, whereas their frustration can result in decreased motivation and mental health challenges. Autonomy refers to the sense of control and self-direction over one's actions. When individuals feel that their choices are self-endorsed and aligned with their values, they are more likely to engage in behaviours that reflect personal growth and self-improvement.

For individuals with offending behaviour, feeling a sense of *autonomy* in their decision-making process is crucial for motivating them towards desistance. *Competence* involves the feeling of effectiveness and capability in one's actions and pursuits. Individuals who experience success and mastery are more motivated to persist in positive behaviours. For offenders, building skills and experiencing achievements in rehabilitation efforts can enhance their sense of competence and support their journey towards desistance. *Relatedness* encompasses the desire for meaningful connections and a sense of belonging with others. Establishing positive relationships and feeling connected to a community can significantly impact an individual's motivation to change. For offenders, feeling supported and understood by others can strengthen their commitment to desisting from crime and integrating into pro-social environments.

Motivation is a critical factor in the desistance process, as it determines an individual's willingness to engage in rehabilitation and make positive changes in their life. According to the Risk-Need-Responsivity (RNR) model (Bonta & Andrews, 2007), addressing motivation is essential for effective interventions. SDT offers valuable insights into ways of fostering motivation by focusing on the fulfilment of autonomy, competence and relatedness. Interventions should aim to enhance autonomy by empowering individuals through involvement in their treatment plans and respecting their personal choices. Encouraging offenders to set their own goals and take ownership of their rehabilitation process can increase their intrinsic motivation to change. Building competence involves providing opportunities for skill development, success and mastery, which can boost offenders' confidence and sustain their motivation. Fostering relatedness requires creating supportive and empathetic relationships with practitioners and peers, which addresses the need for connection and belonging.

Developing positive social connections within the rehabilitation context can enhance motivation and commitment to desistance goals. SDT offers a robust framework for understanding and enhancing motivation in individuals with offending behaviour. By focusing on the fulfilment of autonomy, competence and relatedness, rehabilitation programmes can better support offenders in their journey towards desistance and pro-social living. Integrating SDT principles into intervention strategies can lead to more effective outcomes and foster lasting positive change in individuals' lives.

APPROACH AND AVOIDANCE GOALS IN THE CONTEXT OF DESISTANCE

Goal setting is a critical strategy for individuals who have offended, as it helps redirect their focus towards a positive future and has been shown to effectively reduce recidivism (Fernández-Moreno et al., 2024). Goals can be categorised into approach and avoidance types, each playing a distinct role in shaping behaviour and motivation. Approach goals focus on attaining positive outcomes and achieving desired states or accomplishments. For people desisting from offending, approach goals might include building a fulfilling career, developing meaningful relationships or engaging in activities that bring joy and satisfaction. These goals are aligned with positive emotions and forward-thinking, which can inspire and sustain motivation. For instance, envisioning a future filled with purpose and pleasure can foster hope and optimism, crucial for long-term desistance. On the other hand, avoidance goals are centred on evading negative outcomes or pain. Individuals often set these goals to prevent unpleasant situations or to escape from distress. In the context of offending behaviour, avoidance goals might involve steering clear of situations that could trigger a relapse into criminal activity or substance abuse. While avoidance goals can be practical for immediate harm reduction, relying solely on them may not address underlying issues or promote long-term well-being. To successfully transition away from offending behaviour, it is essential to balance both approach and avoidance goals. Replacing harmful behaviours with constructive alternatives requires not only avoiding negative triggers but also actively pursuing positive experiences and growth. For example, while avoiding substance abuse is crucial, cultivating a sense of purpose and engaging in fulfilling activities can help individuals maintain their commitment to change.

Developing hope for a better future can serve as a powerful approach goal, helping individuals envision and work towards a life free from offending. In tandem with hope, learning self-soothing techniques through compassion training can replace the need for unhealthy coping mechanisms such as drugs or alcohol. Compassion training helps individuals manage distress and fosters emotional resilience, which is crucial for maintaining progress, preventing relapse and developing healthy thinking patterns. Adopting healthy and compassionate thinking styles is linked to improved well-being and pro-social behaviours (Neff et al., 2007; Zeng et al., 2022). Developing a compassionate mind can strengthen positive emotions and foster pro-social behaviours, creating a supportive framework for achieving both approach and avoidance goals. Compassionate thinking also aids in cultivating empathy and effective communication skills, which are vital for building positive relationships and integrating into society. Integrating approach and avoidance goals into the desistance process can guide individuals towards a balanced and fulfilling life. By focusing on positive aspirations, learning healthy coping strategies and maintaining physical well-being, individuals can foster lasting change and reduce the likelihood of returning to offending behaviour.

OFFENDER FLOURISHING, WELL-BEING AND CRIMINAL THINKING STYLES

Flourishing is characterised by optimal well-being across the dimensions of the PERMA model. When individuals are flourishing, they experience high levels of well-being and have a robust active soothing and drive system (Gilbert, 2009). This state is achieved through intentional actions that enhance overall well-being. Conversely, those who are languishing experience low levels of well-being, which may manifest as distress, low mood and a general sense of emptiness. While languishing itself is not classified as a mental health disorder, it is a precursor to conditions such as depression and low mood (Giblett & Hodgins, 2023).

In the context of offending behaviour, flourishing is associated with finding meaning and purpose in life, positive identity change, self-control, forgiveness and accountability (Jang et al., 2023), whereas individuals who struggle with low well-being (languishing) may engage in criminal activities as a means of coping or escaping their malaise and impact of Adverse Childhood Experiences (ACEs) (Ford et al., 2020). Research by Wissing et al. (2021) found that individuals who are languishing tend to focus on self-oriented goals and are motivated by hedonic happiness, which is centred on immediate pleasure and personal satisfaction. In contrast, those who are flourishing are more inclined towards eudemonic goals, which emphasise contributing to the greater good and fostering meaningful connections with others.

BROADEN AND BUILD THEORY

The Broaden and Build theory, proposed by Fredrickson (1998, 2001), extends the understanding of positive emotions beyond momentary happiness. According to this theory, positive emotions expand our thought-action repertoire, enabling us to explore a wider range of solutions to problems and creating an upward spiral of positivity and well-being. For example, joy encourages play and exploration, curiosity drives learning and growth and love fosters connection and relationship building. These positive emotions broaden our cognitive and behavioural responses, helping us to develop personal resources and build social connections. In contrast, negative emotions such as fear, anger and hate narrow our thought-action repertoire, limiting our responses to basic fight-or-flight reactions (Fredrickson, 2004). When individuals are threatened or anxious, their focus tends to be on immediate survival, often leading to aggressive or defensive behaviours. Positive emotions, by broadening our perspectives, enable us to consider a variety of actions and opportunities for conflict resolution and personal development. This broadening effect helps build personal and social resources, which can be crucial for personal growth and the formation of supportive relationships.

This concept aligns with the emotional regulation system in Compassion-Focused Therapy (CFT), where the development of the soothing system facilitates positive change and enhances our ability to manage and respond to challenging situations effectively (Gilbert, 2009). By cultivating positive emotions and building resources through pro-social behaviours and supportive relationships, individuals can foster a state of flourishing that supports their journey towards desistance and improved well-being.

SKILLS AND STRENGTHS OF POSITIVE PSYCHOLOGY TO AID DESISTANCE

Developing positive strengths and qualities is crucial for offenders aiming to desist from criminal behaviour and integrate successfully into society. These skills and strengths can be categorised into four main areas: releasing the past, overcoming challenges, imagining a positive future and enhancing life enjoyment. Positive Psychology offers a range of interventions to support these areas, including practices like forgiveness, hope, optimism, mindsets, savouring, gratitude and leveraging virtues and character strengths.

Forgiveness

Forgiveness can significantly impact an offender's well-being and behaviour. The process of forgiveness involves shifting one's thoughts, feelings and behaviours towards others, either those who have caused harm or oneself. When attacked, whether verbally or physically, our threat response system can drive us towards seeking revenge or withdrawing. Forgiveness helps to transform this response into more pro-social behaviour. Research indicates that forgiving others and oneself can reduce negative emotions and promote psychological healing (McCullough & Witvliet, 2002). Self-forgiveness is a slow and challenging process that requires self-compassion to manage feelings of shame and guilt but can have a significant impact on offender well-being, help them cope with prison and create new life narrative (Moniz et al., 2024). This process can mitigate the long-lasting effects of past wrongs and support a more positive outlook.

Hope

Hope is a critical factor in facilitating change and supporting individuals who are imprisoned. It is particularly effective in adverse situations where it can foster optimism and resilience. High levels of hope are associated with better outcomes in desistance, including the likelihood of avoiding re-offending (Martin & Stermac, 2010) and the need to build a better future and end suffering for self and others among people in prisons (Laursen, 2023). Hope helps individuals reconstruct their identities, seek professional help, build positive relationships and find meaning in their lives. It can be cultivated through community relationships and reflecting on past moments of hope that led to positive changes (Atherton et al., 2022).

Optimism

Both dispositional and learned optimism contribute to improved well-being and are beneficial for desistance. Dispositional optimism refers to the general expectation that good things will happen in life (Carver & Scheier, 2023). In contrast, learned optimism involves altering one's explanatory style to view challenges as temporary and external rather than permanent and personal. This shift in mindset can positively impact motivation and resilience and is stronger when a desister has denser pro-social networks (Nolet et al., 2022). By challenging pessimistic thoughts and adopting a more optimistic outlook, individuals can enhance their ability to cope with setbacks and pursue positive change.

Mindsets

Mindsets, particularly the distinction between fixed and growth mindsets, affect motivation and the ability to overcome challenges (Dweck, 1999). A growth mindset fosters the belief that abilities and intelligence can be developed through effort, while a fixed mindset leads to a belief in static abilities. Those with a growth mindset are more likely to persist through difficulties and view failures as opportunities for learning (Burnette et al., 2023). Encouraging a growth mindset can be supported through educational and technological interventions that build resilience and facilitate skill acquisition and is associated with a positive approach to rehabilitation (Hoyt et al., 2022). Wong (2022) also proposes that a positive suffering mindset (PSM) is needed to overcome suffering and flourish. He also suggests that there are many overlapping mindsets that are key to this and help build positive mental health. In addition to a growth mindset that enables us to grow stronger in the face of adversity, Wong (Wong & Gonot-Schoupinsky, 2024) refers to the following mindsets:

- The mindful mindset helps us see things as they are rather than how we would like them to be.

- The meaning mindset encourages us to see and find the meaning in all situations so that we can grow from them.

- The dialectical mindset calls on us to see the balance in life and the full range of our experiences.

- The resilient mindset teaches us how to learn from and overcome our suffering.

- The self-transcendent mindset refers to the belief that we can overcome obstacles in our way.

Savouring

Savouring involves a mindful appreciation of positive experiences and sur-roundings. For individuals recently released from prison, savouring can enhance the enjoyment of newfound freedom and help shift focus from past hardships to present joys. This practice involves present-moment awareness and appreciation, contributing to a cognitive shift from negative to positive self-talk, and can have a positive impact on the well-being of people who have offended (Fourie & Koen, 2018). By practising savouring, individuals can enhance their positive experiences and cultivate a pro-social identity.

Gratitude

Gratitude, both as an emotional state and a trait, plays a significant role in improving well-being and fostering pro-social behaviour. Expressing gratitude can enhance positive emotions and reduce aggression by increasing appreci-ation for life's positives (Danioni et al., 2023). Techniques for fostering grat-itude include reflecting on things one is grateful for, counting blessings and expressing thanks to those who have positively influenced one's life. These practices can improve social relationships and support positive reintegration into society (Huynh et al., 2015).

Virtues and Character Strengths

Positive Psychology emphasises the importance of character strengths and virtues in achieving personal goals and fostering pro-social behaviour. According to the Values in Action (VIA) classification system, there are six principal virtues and twenty-four-character strengths that can be leveraged for personal development and achieving goals (see Table 1). These virtues and

Table 1. Character Strengths and Virtues.

Wisdom	Courage	Humanity	Justice	Temperance	Transcendence
Creativity	Bravery	Kindness	Fairness	Forgiveness	Appreciation of beauty and excellence
Curiosity	Honesty	Love	Leadership	Humility	Gratitude
Judgement	Perseverance	Social intelligence	Teamwork	Prudence	Hope
Love of learning	Zest			Self-regulation	Humour
Perspective					Spirituality

strengths include attributes such as courage, justice, temperance and wisdom, which can support individuals in their journey towards desistance and flourishing, and are presented in the table below. By focusing on these positive psychological skills and strengths, individuals who have offended can improve their well-being, enhance their ability to cope with challenges and successfully transition to a pro-social life.

CHARACTER STRENGTHS AND THEIR ROLE IN DESISTANCE

Character strengths are integral to Positive Psychology and play a significant role in promoting well-being, resilience and personal growth. For individuals who have offended, understanding and utilising these strengths can be transformative. Character strengths help in identifying who we are, enhancing our well-being and contributing positively to the collective good. They also support mental and physical health, offer resilience in the face of past traumas and foster a sense of meaning in life (Park & Peterson, 2008).

THE IMPACT OF CHARACTER STRENGTHS ON OFFENDER WELL-BEING

For offenders, character strengths can be particularly meaningful. They provide a framework for understanding personal attributes and applying them constructively, which is essential for achieving desistance. For instance, research shows that men convicted of sexual offences demonstrated increased accountability and self-awareness after engaging with the VIA Character Strengths Survey. This process helped them recognise and apply their strengths in positive ways, contributing to post-traumatic growth and a deeper understanding of their needs (Miner, 2021).

VERSATILITY OF CHARACTER STRENGTHS

Character strengths are versatile and applicable across different timeframes, past, present and future. Reflecting on past experiences where strengths were utilised to overcome adversity can provide valuable insights. For example, recalling how courage helped navigate previous challenges can inspire current efforts towards desistance. Similarly, identifying strengths in the present can aid in beginning the journey of desistance, and envisioning how these strengths can be leveraged in the future helps in setting and achieving long-term goals.

Application to the past: Reflecting on past instances where one's strengths were effectively used to overcome challenges can reinforce positive behaviour patterns and provide motivation. This reflection helps individuals recognise their capacity for resilience and problem-solving.

Application to the present: Identifying and actively using character strengths in current situations supports immediate changes in behaviour and attitude. For example, applying strengths such as perseverance and creativity can facilitate effective engagement in pro-social activities and rehabilitation efforts.

Application to the future: Envisioning how to use character strengths to achieve future goals promotes a forward-looking mindset. It encourages individuals to plan and aspire towards positive outcomes, leveraging their strengths to build a better future.

SIGNATURE STRENGTHS AND OPTIMAL UTILISATION

Understanding and applying signature strengths, those that are central to one's identity and most naturally expressed, can greatly enhance well-being and effectiveness in achieving desistance. Signature strengths are unique to each individual and include attributes like courage, honesty and kindness. Utilising these strengths in meaningful ways can boost self-esteem, foster positive relationships and contribute to overall life satisfaction. An awareness of the 'Golden Mean', overuse and underuse of strengths can lead to the expression of the right strengths, in the right situation and to the right degree. Interventions such as strengths spotting, feedback from others and mindful awareness can be utilised when working with offenders to assist in the pursuit of optimal strengths use (Niemiec, 2019).

- *Self-awareness:* Recognising one's character strengths through tools like the VIA Survey enables individuals to understand their core attributes and how these can be applied in various contexts.

- *Strengths-based interventions:* Developing interventions that focus on leveraging these strengths can lead to more effective rehabilitation and personal growth. For example, using creativity in problem-solving or leveraging leadership qualities to guide others in a positive direction can be powerful.

- *Strengths-based goals:* Setting goals that align with one's strengths ensures that efforts are in harmony with personal values and capabilities, leading to greater fulfilment and success.

By focusing on character strengths, individuals who have offended can enhance their personal development, improve their well-being and contribute positively to society. This strengths-based approach not only helps in the journey towards desistance but also in thriving as non-offender members of the community.

CONCLUSION

In this chapter, the author has explored how Positive Psychology offers both theoretical and practical tools to assist individuals who have offended in their journey towards change. By embracing positive psychological principles, individuals can be supported to find hope for the future, make sense of their past and discover motivation in the present. Positive Psychology extends beyond merely achieving a 'good life' and argues that the pursuit of a 'meaningful and happy life' is a crucial component of flourishing and sustained well-being. This approach emphasises that while a good life is important, true flourishing involves integrating positive emotions, engagement, relationships, meaning and accomplishments, concepts central to the PERMA model.

Compassion further enhances the benefits of Positive Psychology by helping individuals reconcile with their past, embrace their strengths and build a life imbued with meaning and purpose. Compassion-based practices, such as self-compassion and forgiveness, align with Positive Psychology principles to facilitate personal growth and resilience. The growing body of literature supporting Positive Psychology interventions for individuals who have offended underscores the value of incorporating these strategies into desistance models. This chapter has highlighted various practical approaches, such as hope, optimism, savouring, gratitude and the application of character strengths, that are instrumental in fostering positive change and personal development.

In summary, Positive Psychology provides a comprehensive framework for supporting individuals in their efforts to move beyond past offending behaviours. Focusing on meaningful goals, cultivating strengths and integrating compassionate practices helps individuals achieve lasting positive change and contribute positively to society.

REFERENCES

Atherton, S., Knight, V., & van Barthold, B. C. (2022). Penal arts interventions and hope: Outcomes of arts-based projects in prisons and community settings. *The Prison Journal, 102*(2), 217–236.

Bonta, J., & Andrews, D. A. (2007). Risk-need-responsivity model for offender assessment and rehabilitation. *Rehabilitation, 6*(1), 1–22.

Burnette, J. L., Billingsley, J., Banks, G. C., Knouse, L. E., Hoyt, C. L., Pollack, J. M., & Simon, S. (2023). A systematic review and meta-analysis of growth mindset interventions: For whom, how, and why might such interventions work? *Psychological Bulletin, 149*(3–4), 174.

Carver, C. S., & Scheier, M. F. (2023). Optimism. In F. Maggino (Ed.), *Encyclopaedia of quality of life and well-being research* (pp. 4849–4854). Springer. https://doi.org/10.1007/978-3-031-17299-1_2018

Csikszentmihalyi, M. (2002). *Flow: The classic work on how to achieve happiness*. Harper & Row.

Danioni, F., Paleari, F. G., Pelucchi, S., Lombrano, M. R., Lumera, D., & Regalia, C. (2023). Gratitude, forgiveness, and anger: Resources and risk factors for Italian prison inmates. *International Journal of Offender Therapy and Comparative Criminology, 67*(2–3), 207–223.

Dweck, C. S. (1999). *Self-theories: Their role in motivation, personality, and development*. Taylor and Francis/Psychology Press.

Fernández-Moreno, Á., Roncero, D., & Moreno-Fernández, R. D. (2024). A new approach to urinalysis: Effectiveness of a contingency management program among adolescent offenders in Spain. *Frontiers in Psychology, 15*, 1364967.

Ford, K., Bellis, M. A., Hughes, K., Barton, E. R., & Newbury, A. (2020). Adverse childhood experiences: A retrospective study to understand their associations with lifetime mental health diagnosis, self-harm or suicide attempt, and current low mental wellbeing in a male Welsh prison population. *Health & Justice, 8*, 1–13.

Fourie, M. E., & Koen, V. (2018). South African female offenders' experiences of the Sycamore Tree Project with strength-based activities. *International Journal of Restorative Justice, 1*, 57.

Fredrickson, B. L. (1998). What good are positive emotions? *Review of General Psychology, 2*(3), 300–319.

Fredrickson, B. L. (2001). The role of positive emotions in positive psychology: The broaden-and-build theory of positive emotions. *American Psychologist, 56*(3), 218.

Fredrickson, B. L. (2004). The broaden–and–build theory of positive emotions. *Philosophical Transactions of the Royal Society of London. Series B: Biological Sciences, 359*(1449), 1367–1377.

Giblett, A., & Hodgins, G. (2023). Flourishing or languishing? The relationship between mental health, health locus of control and generalised self-efficacy. *Psychological Reports, 126*(1), 94–116.

Gilbert, P. (2009). Introducing compassion-focused therapy. *Advances in Psychiatric Treatment, 15*(3), 199–208.

Hoyt, C. L., d'Almeida, A., Forsyth, R. B., & Burnette, J. L. (2022). Mindsets of criminality: Predicting punitive and rehabilitative attitudes. *Psychology, Crime and Law*, 1–18.

Huynh, K. H., Hall, B., Hurst, M. A., & Bikos, L. H. (2015). Evaluation of the positive re-entry in corrections program: A positive psychology intervention with prison inmates. *International Journal of Offender Therapy and Comparative Criminology, 59*(9), 1006–1023.

Jang, S. J., Johnson, B. R., Anderson, M. L., & Booyens, K. (2023). Religion and rehabilitation in Colombian and South African prisons: A human flourishing approach. *International Criminal Justice Review*, 33(3), 225–252.

Laursen, J. (2023). Radical hope and processes of becoming: Examining short-term prisoners' imagined futures in England, Wales and Norway. *Theoretical Criminology*, 27(1), 48–65.

Martin, K., & Stermac, L. (2010). Measuring hope: Is hope related to criminal behaviour in offenders? *International Journal of Offender Therapy and Comparative Criminology*, 54(5), 693–705.

Maruna, S. (2001). *Making good* (Vol. 86). American Psychological Association.

Maslow, A. H. (1954). *Motivation and personality*. Harper & Row, Publishers.

McCullough, M. E., & Witvliet, C. V. (2002). The psychology of forgiveness. In C. R. Snyder (Ed.), *Handbook of positive psychology* (pp. 446–458). Oxford University Press.

McNeill, F., & Schinkel, M. (2024). Tertiary or relational desistance: Contested belonging. *International Journal of Criminal Justice*, 6(1), 47–74.

Miner, T. A. (2021). *Exploring the role of core positive selves with men convicted of child sexual offenses: A character strengths initiative*. The University of New Mexico.

Moniz, J., Nunes, V., & Cunha, C. (2024). Forgiveness and rehabilitation of Portuguese incarcerated individuals: What do they think about forgiveness? *Journal of Offender Rehabilitation*, 63(5), 328–346. https://doi.org/10.1080/10509674.2024.2353568

Neff, K. D., Rude, S. S., & Kirkpatrick, K. L. (2007). An examination of self-compassion in relation to positive psychological functioning and personality traits. *Journal of Research in Personality*, 41(4), 908–916.

Niemiec, R. M. (2019). Finding the golden mean: The overuse, underuse, and optimal use of character strengths. *Counselling Psychology Quarterly*, 32(3–4), 453–471. https://doi.org/10.1080/09515070.2019.1617674

Nolet, A. M., Charette, Y., & Mignon, F. (2022). The effect of prosocial and antisocial relationships structure on offenders' optimism towards desistance. *Canadian Journal of Criminology and Criminal Justice*, 64(2), 59–81.

Olson, J., Martin, R. L., & Connell, N. M. (2021). Satisfaction with life and crime: Testing the link. *Psychology, Crime and Law, 27*(7), 631–655.

Park, N., & Peterson, C. (2008). Positive psychology and character strengths: Application to strengths-based school counseling. *Professional School Counseling, 12*(2), 2156759X0801200214.

Peterson, C. (2008). What is positive psychology, and what is it not. *Psychology Today, 16.*

Ronel, N. (2015). How can criminology (and victimology) become positive? In N. Ronel & D. Segev (Eds.), *Positive criminology* (pp. 13–31). Routledge.

Ryan, R. M., & Deci, E. L. (2000). Self-determination theory and the facilitation of intrinsic motivation, social development, and well-being. *American Psychologist, 55*(1), 68–78.

Seligman, M. E. P. (2002). *Authentic happiness.* Simon & Shuster Inc.

Seligman, M. E. P. (2011). *Flourish: A visionary new understanding of happiness and well-being.* Atria Books.

Seligman, M. E. P. (2019). Positive psychology: A personal history. *Annual Review of Clinical Psychology, 15,* 1–23.

Wissing, M. P., Schutte, L., Liversage, C., Entwisle, B., Gericke, M., & Keyes, C. (2021). Important goals, meanings, and relationships in flourishing and languishing states: Towards patterns of well-being. *Applied Research in Quality of Life, 16*(2), 573–609.

Wong, P. T. P. (2022). The best possible life in a troubled world: The seven principles of self-transcendence. *Positive Psychology in Counseling and Education, 1,* 1–24.

Wong, P. T., & Gonot-Schoupinsky, F. (2024). Mental health and meaning: A positive autoethnographic case study of Paul Wong. *Mental Health and Social Inclusion.* https://doi.org/10.1108/MHSI-06-2024-0092

Zeng, P., Nie, J., Geng, J., Wang, H., Chu, X., Qi, L., Wang, P., & Lei, L. (2022). Self-compassion and subjective well-being: A moderated mediation model of online prosocial behavior and gratitude. *Psychology in the Schools, 60*(6), 2041–2057. https://doi.org/10.1002/pits.22849

6

DESISTANCE CAPITAL

ABSTRACT

In this chapter, I briefly examine the theories of desistance and capital to explore how they can be integrated into the concept of desistance capital. Desistance capital is the collection of resources and forms of capital that individuals leverage when pursuing a life free from offending. This chapter examines how individuals who have offended might possess significant amounts of capital that, while potentially beneficial, are often used in ways that reinforce anti-social behaviours rather than fostering pro-social outcomes. The discussion highlights the crucial distinction between anti-social and pro-social uses of capital and underscores the necessity of understanding this difference to effectively support desistance. This chapter also provides an overview of various forms of capital, namely human capital, social capital, justice capital and community capital, exploring how each type can facilitate and obstruct the desistance process. By analysing these different forms of capital, this chapter aims to offer insights into how individuals transitioning away from offending can utilise their resources more constructively, ultimately enhancing their chances of achieving lasting change and integration into society.

Keywords: Desistance; capital; assisted desistance; theories; personal perspectives of desistance

DEFINING DESISTANCE

Desistance, in its most basic sense, means to stop or cease a particular behaviour. Although not commonly used by those who have offended themselves, the term 'desistance' is prevalent in probation services and the criminal justice system to describe the process of ending criminal behaviour (Maruna & Mann, 2019). Desistance can be understood in two primary ways. First, it can refer to a definitive end point where an individual is recognised as having ceased their offending behaviour entirely (i.e. they have 'desisted'). Second, it can be seen as an ongoing process through which individuals who have offended work to create a new, crime-free life for themselves, often described as 'making good' (Maruna, 2001). Given the complexities and challenges associated with stopping offending, desistance is sometimes defined not only as complete cessation of offending but also as a significant reduction in both the frequency and severity of criminal behaviour (Laub & Sampson, 2001). Additionally, another perspective defines desistance in terms of time; for instance, an individual might be considered a desister if they have refrained from offending for several years and are statistically indistinguishable from the general population of non-offenders (Bushway et al., 2001). However, this approach raises challenges related to accurately identifying who truly falls into the category of 'non-offender', as offences often go undetected and are recorded only when individuals are apprehended. A common benchmark for considering someone as having desisted is a period of seven years without offending (Kurlychek et al., 2007). This estimate is widely accepted, though it can be somewhat arbitrary and may not account for the individual variations in the desistance process. The concept of desistance, therefore, involves both the practicalities of reducing criminal behaviour and the subjective experience of personal change and societal reintegration (Farrall & Shapland, 2022).

THEORIES OF DESISTANCE

Desistance theory seeks to explain how individuals eventually cease their offending behaviours, building upon insights from life-course criminology and the age-crime curve. This curve suggests that criminal activity typically begins in early adolescence, peaks in late teenage years and generally declines as individuals mature, often reaching near-zero levels around age 45 (Gottfredson & Hirschi, 1983). Contributing factors to this decline include negative peer influences, rebellion against authority, shifts in priorities towards employment and stable relationships and life stability resulting from meaningful work and supportive partnerships. However, this perspective has been critiqued for its external locus of control, where desistance is seen as dependent on external factors like employment and marriage. If these external factors are lost, it may increase the risk of re-offending.

The age-crime curve, according to Gottfredson and Hirschi (1983), is universal and consistent, suggesting that everyone, regardless of context or offence type, will eventually stop offending as they age. Yet, this model does not fully explain why or how desistance occurs, leading to a dichotomy between theories emphasising personal agency and those focusing on social systems and structures. This dichotomy reflects deeper philosophical debates about determinism versus free will and individual control over life choices.

One prominent structural theory is Sampson and Laub's (1993) age-graded theory of informal social control. This theory posits that informal social controls, such as stable employment, marriage and parenthood, provide stability and adherence to social norms that facilitate desistance. The emphasis is on significant life events and social connections which, like Fredrickson's (2004) Broaden and Build theory, expand an individual's social repertoire. Some theories view individuals as bound by social forces and cultural inhibitors, while others see them as empowered but constrained by their social situations (Farrall & Bowling, 1999). This perspective suggests that individuals actively work towards change, either by transforming their self-concept or by addressing dissatisfaction with their criminal behaviour and fear of future repercussions (Giordano et al., 2002; Maruna, 2001; Paternoster & Bushway, 2009).

Giordano et al. (2002) propose a four-stage theory of cognitive transformation in desistance: (1) Openness to change, (2) exposure to hooks for change, (3) the cognitive appeal of a replacement self and (4) transformation in views of deviance. The first stage involves recognising the need for change and a willingness to pursue it. In the second stage, individuals must encounter opportunities that facilitate change. The third and fourth stages involve envisioning a non-criminal future and reinterpreting past criminal behaviour as undesirable and irrelevant to their new identity.

Maruna's (2001) Liverpool Desistance Study highlights the role of personal agency in desistance. His research revealed that individuals who successfully desisted from crime often developed a pro-social identity supported by a 'redemption script' rather than a 'condemnation script'. Redemption scripts involve viewing oneself as fundamentally good despite past criminal behaviour, with support from society aiding this positive transformation. In contrast, condemnation scripts involve blaming external factors and perpetuating an external locus of control, often resulting in continued offending. Helping individuals adopt a redemption script and fostering their self-belief and responsibility are crucial for successful desistance and can be likened to developing a compassionate self.

The impact of social identity and societal perceptions is also significant. Ex-offenders often face stigma and are labelled negatively due to their criminal pasts. This negative labelling can reinforce a condemnation narrative, undermining hope and increasing recidivism risks. Conversely, those with a redemption script actively work to build positive identities, such as being a good parent or a responsible worker, which enhances community support and fosters long-term desistance. Maruna (2001) found that individuals who could make sense of their past, find purpose in their lives and have a clear vision for the future were more successful in desisting from crime.

Interactionist approaches, which combine social contextual factors with individual choices, offer additional insights into the desistance process. These approaches highlight the dynamic interplay between personal agency and social influences, illustrating that desistance is not a straightforward or linear process but a complex journey shaped by individual decisions and external circumstances (King, 2014). Understanding desistance requires acknowledging this complexity and providing supportive environments facilitating personal transformation and reintegration.

THE STAGES OF DESISTANCE

Desistance is often conceptualised through stages that highlight different aspects of the process. Initially, Farrell and Maruna (2004) categorised desistance into two main stages: primary and secondary desistance. Primary desistance refers to the cessation of the offending behaviour itself. At this stage, the focus is on the absence of criminal acts, which might be temporary or long term. Secondary desistance, on the other hand, involves a more profound transformation, where individuals actively reshape their identity away from being an offender to becoming a non-offender. This stage emphasises the importance of adopting new self-concepts and discarding old labels associated with criminal behaviour.

King (2013) challenges the idea that changes in identity occur only after a period of non-offending. Instead, he argues that shifts in identity can start before any behavioural change. It is plausible that identity and behaviour changes co-occur, reflecting an internal struggle as individuals wrestle with their past selves and their desired future selves and acceptance into society.

This internal conflict underscores the need for compassionate and hopeful support in crafting a new identity.

McNeill (2016) expanded this framework by introducing a third stage: tertiary desistance. This stage involves societal acceptance and a sense of belonging after desistance has been achieved. Tertiary desistance focuses on how individuals are perceived by society and their integration into the community as positive contributors. This stage reflects the importance of public opinion and the role of societal structures in removing barriers to desistance, thereby supporting individuals in maintaining their crime-free status and enhancing their social and community capital.

The desistance process is inherently complex and often involves lapses and relapses, particularly for individuals with long-term offending histories. Various factors influence the trajectory of desistance, including the individual's criminal achievements and their cognitive skills. Those with extensive criminal careers might require time and cognitive support to facilitate identity change, whereas individuals with less severe criminal histories might face different challenges. Successful offenders, such as high-level drug traffickers, may not view themselves as criminals but rather as business operators, which influences their desistance process (Vidal et al., 2020). Understanding these diverse self-perceptions can inform tailored support for individuals in their desistance journey.

PERSONAL PERSPECTIVE ON DESISTANCE

From a personal perspective, desisting is both a process and an end-point. The end-point is the goal one hopes to reach where they have stopped and does not desire to return to offending. The process is the steps taken from that decisive point where the decision to stop offending is made and efforts put in place to commit to the choice to not offend. I try to avoid the term 'go straight' here because it implies that desistance is a linear process when we know that this is not the case. It can also be self-stigmatising because it implies that we are bent out of shape because we have offended. Because of the ongoing process, it is more a definition of desisting rather than desisted. We are all desisting from offending just as we are all trying to be a good person. Even now, as a person with a PhD and the title Doctor, am I still considered a desister because the potential for offending is always there, or have I desisted because I choose never to offend again and have not done for a lot longer than seven years? To put a time frame on desistance is to add yet another barrier to someone trying to make changes to their life and stop offending. In the same way, we all make mistakes and try not to repeat those same mistakes. We do our best not to be held by them and consider them to be a part of our past. Even though we are punished for our offences within a set period, the stigma imposed on us by others lasts much longer. We are limited on where we can go and what countries we can visit, in some cases for life, regardless of how much we have changed since our conviction. Society does not hold us accountable for all our transgressions in the same way it does for our offences, nor does it measure or time us on these changes in behaviour. One is just easier to stigmatise than the other because it involves breaking the law, even though both can be judged the same. Still, it is difficult to maintain the hope needed to desist when faced with multiple social and justice barriers. At the end of the day, you are the only one who really knows when you've desisted.

Nevertheless, desistance is a process, a journey of self-development, disclosure and discovery about whom we are, our place in the world and the potential we have within us to make good for ourselves and others. Like everything else in life, it is neither straightforward nor easy. Desistance is not something that cannot be bound by time or space because the nature of offending behaviour is more complex than that. It is non-linear and, like the process of time, needs to be explored by standing back and looking at the past, present and future as one. Rather than go straight, we need to go North and find the guiding star that pulls us forward, discovering who we really are and want to be. And just like any journey of discovery, we must remind ourselves that the path towards redemption is seldom straight, but that salvation lies at the end of a long and winding road. And along that journey, we need others to assist us, whether that is through direct or indirect support by removing the barriers that stand in our way, and it is there where we find the true meaning of desistance.

DESISTANCE VERSUS REHABILITATION

Rehabilitation traditionally follows a medical model, treating offending behaviour as a condition to be fixed through interventions imposed by professionals. This approach implies that individuals are 'broken' and need correction. In contrast, desistance theory emphasises self-directed change and personal agency. Maruna (2016) suggests that individuals either desist on their own accord or through formal rehabilitation efforts. However, desistance can also be supported through various means, including compassionate guidance, hope, optimism and the removal of barriers. Desistance represents a complex, non-linear process that combines internal motivation and external support. It involves both behavioural change and a redefinition of identity, often requiring supportive social environments to facilitate long-term success. Unlike rehabilitation, which often focuses on fixing problems, desistance emphasises personal growth, agency and the integration of individuals into the community as contributing members.

HELPING THE PROCESS: ASSISTED DESISTANCE

Assisted desistance encompasses the range of support that organisations and practitioners can provide to individuals seeking to cease offending and reintegrate into society (Maruna, 2010). This support involves both practical assistance and the fostering of positive, encouraging relationships that inspire optimism and hope for the future (Chouhy et al., 2020). The support can be categorised into direct and indirect forms. Direct support includes tangible help such as securing job opportunities, providing housing or offering counselling. For instance, a justice practitioner might assist an individual in finding employment or accessing rehabilitation services. Indirect support, on the other hand, refers to less overt forms of assistance. This might include the emotional and psychological impact of family visits or community support, which can motivate an individual to reconsider their behaviour. Assisted desistance can also be classified as formal or informal. Formal support is provided through structured programmes and professional services, including those offered by probation officers, counsellors, and rehabilitation programmes. Informal support comes from community members or peer support groups. For example, volunteers at addiction charities or community organisations in the United Kingdom, like Timpson's, offer informal assistance that plays a crucial role in the desistance process.

Understanding assisted desistance through the concept of capital, referring to the resources and assets available to an individual, can be particularly insightful. This includes human capital, which encompasses the skills, knowledge and experiences that individuals can leverage for positive change. Those with substantial human capital might be better equipped to navigate the desistance process independently. Social capital involves the networks and relationships that provide support and opportunities. This includes family, friends and community connections. Justice capital refers to the resources provided by the criminal justice system, including rehabilitation programmes and supportive interventions. Community capital involves the broader support available within the community, such as local charities and social services.

Research by McNeill et al. (2012) identifies eight principles essential for desistance-focused criminal justice practice. These principles include:

(1) Being realistic about the complexity of the desistance process.

(2) Individualising support.

(3) Building and sustaining hope.

(4) Recognising and developing people's strengths.

(5) Respecting and fostering agency.

(6) Working through relationships.

(7) Developing social and human capital.

(8) Recognising and celebrating progress.

Additionally, a ninth principle is suggested. It is developing compassion directed at oneself and others, including both desisters and practitioners, to support the desistance process. Compassion fosters a supportive environment that enhances resilience and encourages positive change.

Practitioners need to be aware of several factors related to assisted desistance. Early in the desistance journey, individuals often face barriers such as difficulties in leaving behind prior offending lifestyles and adapting to a new identity (Farrall, 2005). Compassionate support is essential in helping individuals navigate these challenges. Post-incarceration trauma and the emotional struggles associated with desisting can also present significant obstacles. Addressing past traumas and providing emotional support can facilitate healing and help individuals overcome these barriers (Towne et al., 2023).

Practical assistance with issues such as housing, financial stability, employment and substance abuse is vital. Practitioners should help individuals set goals, identify resources and develop structured plans to support their desistance. This practical support provides the foundation for building a new identity and achieving successful reintegration into society (King, 2014). Compassionate Mind Training (CMT) can be an effective tool in helping individuals envision a positive future and stay motivated to desist from offending. By demonstrating a genuine, non-judgmental attitude, practitioners can build positive relationships that support individuals in reaching their goals and integrating successfully into society (Villeneuve et al., 2021).

Assisted desistance requires a multifaceted approach that combines practical support with compassionate understanding. Practitioners and organisations play a crucial role in helping individuals navigate the complex journey away from offending, address emotional and practical challenges and build the necessary capital for successful reintegration. The principles of desistance-focused practice, along with an emphasis on compassion, provide a comprehensive framework for supporting individuals in their desistance journey.

CAPITAL THEORY

The concept of capital originates from economics and encompasses various forms of resources and assets that individuals accumulate over time, which enable them to thrive in life. French economist Pierre Bourdieu (1986) described capital as having 'accumulated history' and as a form of effective power that creates differentiation and unequal distribution among groups. Capital can be seen as the resources accrued from previous efforts, which lead to favourable outcomes and influence one's social standing and future opportunities. Different types of capital, personal, social and community can transform into one another. For instance, psychological capital can enhance social capital, and vice versa, thereby benefiting the individual and increasing their overall capital.

Psychological capital, which includes confidence, optimism and resilience, can influence social capital. Positive psychological capital often stems from interactions with parents, caregivers and peers, and investing in this capital can foster the beliefs and confidence necessary to set and achieve higher goals. This, in turn, reinforces psychological capital through positive feedback and support, leading to improved productivity, career opportunities and general well-being. However, psychological or human capital heavily depends on one's social environment and relationships. Individuals from marginalised groups, such as those involved in offending, might lack access to the same level of capital, resulting in unequal distribution among groups. For instance, those with limited psychological capital may have fewer opportunities to achieve their goals, low self-expectations and inadequate role models. This scarcity of resources can create a self-fulfilling prophecy, where individuals internalise a pessimistic view of themselves and their potential, leading to mental health issues, shame, low self-esteem and a sense of helplessness (Dóci et al., 2023). Increasing positive psychological capital can shift this negative mindset, improve overall well-being and enhance social mobility.

DESISTANCE-FOCUSED VS OFFENDING-FOCUSED CAPITAL

While it is crucial to understand the types of capital that support desistance from offending, it is also important to consider the capital that perpetuates offending behaviours. Criminal capital refers to the resources and networks facilitating criminal activities (McCarthy & Hagan, 1995). Just as desistance-focused capital can lead someone away from crime, criminal capital can sustain offending behaviours (Lindegaard & Jacques, 2014). Desistance involves processes and supports that help individuals maintain crime-free behaviour after offending. For effective desistance, a combination of personal agency (human capital) and supportive social networks (social and community capital) is necessary, such as finding stable employment and receiving positive family support (Kay, 2016; McNeill, 2006). Emphasising personal agency alone, without supportive societal structures, can hinder desistance efforts. Improving social capital is one approach to supporting desistance, but it must be approached cautiously. Offenders may already possess social capital, though it might be more anti-social than pro-social. The key to successful desistance is not merely acquiring more capital but reorienting how individuals obtain and utilise capital in their journey away from offending. The nature of their relationships and the time invested in developing both anti-social and pro-social capital significantly impact the outcomes of these interactions (Kay, 2022).

TYPES OF CAPITAL RELEVANT TO OFFENDING AND DESISTANCE

Four key areas of the capital are relevant to understanding offending behaviour and facilitating desistance: human/psychological capital, social capital, justice capital and community capital.

Human/psychological capital: This encompasses the individual's psychological resources, motivational factors, personal skills and sense of identity, related to offending or desistance.

Social capital: This refers to the network of social relationships and connections that can either promote desistance or perpetuate offending behaviours.

Justice capital: This involves the resources and support that justice organisations and their personnel provide, which can either aid or hinder desistance efforts.

Community capital: This includes the broader community resources and opportunities that support either the continuation of offending or the path to desistance.

Understanding how these types of capital interact and influence both offending and desistance is crucial. The Compassionate Positive Applied Strengths-based Solutions (COMPASS) model will provide a more detailed exploration of these areas and their implications for supporting desistance.

CONCLUSION

Desistance presents a more empowering and less stigmatising approach to ceasing offending behaviour, compared to traditional rehabilitation methods. While rehabilitation often implies a problem that needs fixing by suggesting a binary state of 'rehabilitated' or 'not rehabilitated', desistance recognises the journey as a continuous process. This perspective acknowledges that individuals are not merely transitioning from a problem-state but are instead embarking on a dynamic path towards a crime-free life. Desistance involves a complex interplay of personal and social factors, where individuals gradually shift from offending-focused capital to desistance-focused capital. It requires developing human capital, skills, mindset and agency, that empowers individuals to move away from offending. Equally important is fostering social capital, which includes building pro-social relationships and networks, which in turn enhances the community capital and creates a supportive environment for positive change. To effectively support desistance, it is crucial to view capital from a neutral perspective. Capital is not inherently positive or negative; how it is utilised determines its impact. Desistance involves not only acquiring social capital but also reorienting it towards more pro-social uses while managing the balance between pro-social and anti-social capital. Desistance capital, therefore, encapsulates the resources and support systems available to individuals in their journey away from offending. This concept can guide justice professionals and organisations in understanding and providing the necessary support for those desisting from crime. Recognising that this path is complex and non-linear underscores the importance of a structured approach, such as the COMPASS model, to effectively navigate the challenges and nuances of desistance.

REFERENCES

Bourdieu, P. (1986). The forms of capital. In J. Richardson (Ed.), *Handbook of theory and research for the sociology of education* (pp. 241–258). Greenwood.

Bushway, S. D., Piquero, A. R., Broidy, L. M., Cauffman, E., & Mazerolle, P. (2001). An empirical framework for studying desistance as a process. *Criminology*, *39*(2), 491–516.

Chouhy, C., Cullen, F. T., & Lee, H. (2020). A social support theory of desistance. *Journal of Developmental and Life-Course Criminology*, *6*, 204–223.

Dóci, E., Spruyt, B., De Moortel, D., Vanroelen, C., & Hofmans, J. (2023). In search of the social in psychological capital: Integrating psychological capital into a broader capital framework. *Review of General Psychology*, *27*(3), 336–350.

Farrall, S., & Maruna, S. (2004). Desistance-focused criminal justice policy research: Introduction to a special issue on desistance from crime and public policy. *The Howard Journal of Criminal Justice*, *43*(4), 358–367.

Farrall, S. (2005). On the existential aspects of desistance from crime. *Symbolic Interaction*, *28*(3), 367–386.

Farrall, S., & Bowling, B. (1999). Structuration, human development and desistance from crime. *British Journal of Criminology*, *39*(2), 253–268.

Farrall, S., & Shapland, J. (2022). Do the reasons why people desist from crime vary by age, length of offending career or lifestyle factors? *The Howard Journal of Crime and Justice*, *61*(4), 519–539.

Fredrickson, B. L. (2004). The broaden–and–build theory of positive emotions. *Philosophical Transactions of the Royal Society of London. Series B: Biological Sciences*, *359*(1449), 1367–1377.

Giordano, P. C., Cernkovich, S. A., & Rudolph, J. L. (2002). Gender, crime, and desistance: Toward a theory of cognitive transformation. *American Journal of Sociology*, *107*(4), 990–1064.

Gottfredson, M., & Hirschi, T. (1983). Age and the explanation of crime. *American Journal of Sociology*, *89*(3), 552–584.

Kay, C. (2016). Good cop, bad cop, both? Examining the implications of risk-based allocation on the desistance narratives of intensive probationers. *Probation Journal*, *63*(2), 162–168.

Kay, C. (2022). Rethinking social capital in the desistance process: The 'Artful Dodger' complex. *European Journal of Criminology*, *19*(5), 1243–1259.

King, S. (2013). Assisted desistance and experiences of probation supervision. *Probation Journal*, 60(2), 136–151.

King, S. (2014). *Desistance transitions and the impact of probation.* Routledge.

Kurlychek, M. C., Brame, R., & Bushway, S. D. (2007). Enduring risk? Old criminal records and predictions of future criminal involvement. *Crime & Delinquency*, 53(1), 64–83.

Laub, J. H., & Sampson, R. J. (2001). Understanding desistance from crime. *Crime and Justice*, 28, 1–69.

Lindegaard, M. R., & Jacques, S. (2014). Agency as a cause of crime. *Deviant Behavior*, 35(2), 85–100.

Maruna, S. (2001). *Making good* (Vol. 86). American Psychological Association.

Maruna, S. (2010). The desistance paradigm in correctional practice: From programmes to lives. In F. McNeill, P. Raynor, & C. Trotter (Eds.), *Offender supervision: New directions in theory, research and practice* (pp. 65–89). Willan.

Maruna, S. (2016). Desistance and restorative justice: It's now or never. *Restorative Justice*, 4(3), 289–301. https://doi.org/10.1080/20504721.2016.1243853

Maruna, S., & Mann, R. (2019). Learning desistance together. *Journal of Prison Education and Reentry*, 6(1).

McCarthy, B., & Hagan, J. (1995). Getting into street crime: The structure and process of criminal embeddedness. *Social Science Research*, 24(1), 63–95.

McNeill, F. (2006). A desistance paradigm for offender management. *Criminology and Criminal Justice*, 6(1), 39–62.

McNeill, F. (2016). Desistance and criminal justice in Scotland. In H. Croall, G. Mooney, & R. Munro (Eds.), *Crime, justice, and society in Scotland* (pp. 200–216). Routledge.

McNeill, F., Farrall, S., Lightowler, C., & Maruna, S. (2012). *How and why people stop offending: Discovering desistance.* Insights evidence summary to support Social Services in Scotland. Institute for Research and Innovation in Social Services.

Paternoster, R., & Bushway, S. (2009). Desistance and the 'feared self': Toward an identity theory of criminal desistance. *Journal of Criminal Law and Criminology*, 1103–1156.

Sampson, R. J., & Laub, J. H. (1993). *Crime in the making: Pathways and turning points through life*. Harvard University Press.

Towne, K., Campagna, M., Spohn, R., & Richey, A. (2023). "Put it in your toolbox": How vocational programs support formerly incarcerated persons through re-entry. *Crime & Delinquency*, 69(2), 316–341.

Vidal, S., Ouellet, F., & Dubois, M. È. (2020). Walking into the sunset: How criminal achievement shapes the desistance process: Criminal achievement and the desistance process. *Criminal Justice and Behaviour*, 47(11), 1529–1546.

Villeneuve, M. P., Duffour, I., & Farrall, S. (2021). Assisted desistance in formal settings: A scoping review. *The Howard Journal of Crime and Justice*, 60(1), 75–100.

7

BRINGING IT ALL TOGETHER: INTRODUCING THE COMPASS MODEL FOR CRIMINAL AND FORENSIC PSYCHOLOGY

ABSTRACT

This chapter introduces the Compassionate Positive Applied Strengths-based Solutions (COMPASS) model, a new framework designed to guide practitioners and people in criminal and forensic psychology. It begins by outlining the aims and objectives of the model and then details each of its components. This chapter also discusses the model's practical implications, providing examples and suggestions for working with individuals who have offended. The model emphasises a holistic approach, considering the past, present and future in relation to four key areas of capital: human, social, justice and community.

Keywords: Desistance; capital; zero point; past; present; future

THE COMPASSIONATE POSITIVE APPLIED STRENGTHS-BASED SOLUTIONS (COMPASS) MODEL: AN OVERVIEW

Like the navigational tool used by explorers, our moral compass is said to point to the true North, representing what is considered good. When people veer off course, society or even the individuals themselves may view this as inherently bad or indicative of a lacking moral compass. Some believe a person can be born with a faulty moral compass that cannot be fixed, viewing consistent offending behaviour as evidence of an inherent flaw. The moral consequences of this perspective include shame and guilt. Alternatively, some believe that morality is more malleable. According to this view, there are two main reasons we become morally adrift: intrapersonal limitations in our cognitive biases and interpersonal influences from others (Moore & Gino, 2013). Thus, it is not that we lose our compass; rather, it gets knocked out of alignment by forces beyond our awareness.

The COMPASS model serves as both a theoretical framework and a practical guide for practitioners in the criminal justice system. COMPASS stands for Compassionate Positive Applied Strengths-based Solutions. It integrates techniques and interventions from Compassion-Focused Therapy (CFT), positive psychology, scientific understandings of well-being and strengths-based practices to support people desisting from offending. According to the COMPASS model, for positive change to occur, risks and pro-social needs must be addressed across different areas of the capital, facilitated by individualised interventions focused on understanding and motivation for change.

Working on the principle that all people deserve compassion, the COMPASS model embodies and encourages the need for pro-social support. It empowers individuals by steering them towards desistance-focused outcomes rather than dictating specific goals or future desires. Thus, this model works on the principle that collaboration between professional and service users is vital, with compassion as a core link between an anti-social and pro-social identity. Further, it outlines how a compassionate and positive approach can help individuals develop their own pro-social identity by considering their past experiences, traumas and strengthening protective factors.

ASSUMPTIONS OF THE COMPASS MODEL

Drawing inspiration from earlier theories on why people offend, the COMPASS model combines biopsychosocial theories, such as strain theory, biological drivers and cognitive thinking patterns, with evidence-based interventions from CFT and positive psychology. It promotes well-being and flourishing among those desisting from offending. The model assumes that offending arises from an imbalanced emotional regulation system (threat/drive focused), limited access to pro-social resources and capital and a lack of hope and optimism about oneself and one's future. These factors contribute to a belief in a fixed identity and mindset, with offending becoming an unintended consequence. Change, according to the COMPASS model, occurs through a personal decision to desist and the development of a compassionate understanding of past experiences and the strengths needed to navigate the desistance journey.

THE PAST, PRESENT AND FUTURE

A key assumption of the COMPASS model is that to prevent offending behaviour and foster change, an individual's past, present and future should be explored and understood holistically rather than simply being assessed as risks or goods. A compassionate approach is necessary to understand the reasons behind their behaviour, potential risk factors, unresolved traumas, current situation and future goals. Following an assisted desistance approach, a combination of CFT and positive psychology exercises can be applied at each time point to support the individual's journey.

Past (Southern Point – S): The COMPASS model assumes that a person's past experiences and social environment shape their present identity. As we saw in Chapter 2, evidence suggests that there is a significant link between traumatic backgrounds and offending behaviour. Therefore, trauma-informed compassionate understanding of self and others is key to joint discovery between the individual and the practitioner. Drawing on positive psychology, forgiveness is used to help individuals make sense of and release past experiences. Offending behaviour is seen as developing from a combination of psychological, social and biological factors, including tricky brains, emotional regulation issues and a threat-driven system focused on anti-social actions. Formulating a compassionate understanding of past experiences, previous desistance capital, Adverse Childhood Experiences (ACEs), risks, triggers and unintended consequences helps identify adaptive functioning and motivation towards offending. Positive psychological principles such as forgiveness and gratitude can be applied to the past.

Present: The COMPASS model emphasises embracing the present, focusing on how individuals view themselves in the moment. Motivation to change is explored collaboratively, with a focus on current desistance capital and strengths. Grounding techniques from compassion-focused therapy bring attention to the present, providing a starting point for change. Narrative theory and autobiographical stories help individuals answer questions about their journey and future aspirations. Understanding one's past helps shape future identity.

Future (Northern Point – N): The COMPASS model prioritises the individual's goals and future needs. Practitioners guide individuals towards their goals by exploring desistance capital, emotional well-being and practical needs. Changing the narrative script and re-writing the future involves developing the best possible version of oneself. A COMPASS My Alternative Plan (MAP) is created to chart a course, highlighting the capital needed to achieve goals and maintain desistance. Like the Broden and Build theory, mapping your future increases positive emotions and experiences. Virtual reality (VR) research has shown that imagining and interacting with a future self can motivate change and reduce self-defeating behaviours (van Gelder et al., 2022). Focusing on the future helps give the person more control on what they want rather than them give into external forces that sweep them downstream and bash them from rock to rock.

AIMS OF THE COMPASS MODEL

The primary aim of the COMPASS model is to provide a guide for people desisting from offending and practitioners working with them. It aims to address past criminogenic risk factors through a compassionate approach and recognise strengths to develop and achieve future goals through positive psychology interventions. The model seeks to direct individuals towards a crime-free future, improve well-being and reduce the impact of crime on society. It emphasises compassion in understanding and supporting offending behaviour, considering past experiences and biopsychosocial factors as drivers of offending.

Further aims include promoting desistance by reducing risk factors and behaviours associated with offending and improving protective factors and pro-social behaviours. A compassionate understanding of trauma, shame and guilt helps facilitate change and foster well-being. The COMPASS model also supports practitioners, therapists and probation staff in navigating the challenging emotions involved in working with people who have offended.

To summarise, the COMPASS model is a strengths-based, desistance-focused framework grounded in compassion and positive psychology. It offers a holistic approach to understanding and supporting individuals on their journey towards a pro-social life, addressing past, present and future aspects of their lives.

THE COMPASS MODEL IN RELATION TO OTHER MODELS

In this section, examples of the COMPASS model in relation to current models are presented (see Table 2). The COMPASS model provides and alternative approach to supporting people who have offended along their desistance journey.

Table 2. The COMPASS Model in Relation to the RNR and GLM Models.

Risk-Need-Responsivity	COMPASS	Good Lives Model
Anti-social personality traits/ pro-criminal attitudes	Develop compassionate/hopeful thinking patterns/attitudes (human capital, justice capital)	Inner peace, creativity and knowledge

Table 2. (*Continued*)

Risk-Need-Responsivity	COMPASS	Good Lives Model
Social supports for crime. Lack of involvement in pro-social recreation/leisure activities	Avoid anti-social and engage in pro-social activities and groups (social and community capital)	Excellence in play, agency. Pleasure
Inappropriate parenting/familial relationships	Develop and build positive pro-social relationships (social and community capital)	Relatedness and community
Low employment/education	Find meaning in life through work and education (human, social, justice community capital)	Excellence in work
Substance abuse Self-esteem Vague feelings of personal distress	Developing distress tolerance, hope and effective coping (human capital, justice capital)	Spirituality, life
Major mental disorder Physical health	Home – somewhere to live (community capital)	

KEY COMPONENTS OF THE COMPASS MODEL

Develop Compassionate and Hopeful Thinking Patterns (Human Capital)

Pro-social human capital is defined by transforming maladaptive, pro-criminal attitudes into adaptive behaviours and psychological processes that support desistance. This involves developing a compassionate mindset and fostering positive psychological states that encourage pro-social actions, benefiting the individual, the community and society. Understanding past experiences and their impact on behaviour is crucial, as is taking responsibility and finding a positive path away from offending. Key aspects include:

• *Healthy emotional regulation:* Learning to manage emotions constructively.

• *Pro-social identity:* Developing a sense of self that aligns with societal norms and values.

• *Positive outlook:* Maintaining an optimistic view of the future.

• *Strength and courage:* Building resilience to face and overcome challenges.

Avoid Anti-social and Engage in Pro-social Activities and Groups (Social and Community Capital)

Building pro-social social and community capital involves engaging with individuals and groups who are not involved in offending while making efforts to avoid those who are. These relationships reduce the risk of offending and enhance well-being and social connectedness. Activities can include:

- *Work and volunteering:* Participating in paid or voluntary work.

- *Education:* Pursuing educational opportunities.

- *Social environments:* Joining social centres, support groups or places of worship.

- *Community engagement:* Establishing connections in environments that promote pro-social interactions.

- *Reconnecting with non-offending friends:* Strengthening ties with old friends who are not involved in criminal activities.

Develop and Build Positive Pro-social Relationships (Social and Community Capital)

Positive relationships with significant others in the family and extended circle support bridging and bonding capital. This also extends to developing pro-social relationships through community social establishments that promote cultural relations and supportive environments. Efforts should focus on:

- *Family and extended circle:* Strengthening ties with supportive family members and friends.

- *Community social establishments:* Engaging in community centres and cultural organisations that foster supportive relationships.

Find Meaning in Life and Achievement in Work and Education (Human, Social, Community Capital)

Achieving personal goals and utilising skills and abilities are central to finding meaning in life. Guidance should be provided to develop human capital that opens access to other capital areas. For example:

- *Education and training:* Gaining qualifications that lead to further educational or employment opportunities.

- *Work and career development:* Building a career that aligns with personal goals and societal contributions.

- *Social connections:* Establishing connections that support professional and personal growth.

Develop Distress Tolerance, Hope and Effective Coping (Human Capital)

Developing a compassionate mind increases distress tolerance and can assist with issues like substance abuse, self-esteem and mental and physical health. This fosters a collaborative therapeutic relationship between the person desisting and the practitioner. Key elements include:

- *Compassionate mind:* Enhancing empathy and self-compassion.

- *Distress tolerance:* Building the ability to endure and manage emotional distress.

- *Hope and optimism:* Encouraging a hopeful and positive outlook on the future.

- *Effective coping strategies:* Developing tools and techniques to manage stress and challenges constructively.

The COMPASS model integrates these components to support individuals desisting from offending. By fostering compassionate and hopeful thinking patterns, engaging in pro-social activities, building positive relationships, finding meaningful achievements and developing effective coping strategies, the model provides a comprehensive framework for practitioners and individuals to collaboratively work towards a crime-free and fulfilling life.

THE ZERO POINT AND RATIONALE FOR INTEGRATING COMPASSION AND POSITIVE PSYCHOLOGY WITH DESISTANCE CAPITAL

Positive psychology and compassion are both proven methodologies for improving the well-being of offenders, altering criminal thinking and reducing reoffending rates. Each approach has a robust evidence base supporting the interventions used in both prison and community settings. However, their combined application represents a novel, integrative approach. Compassion focuses on addressing shame and guilt associated with past experiences and offending behaviour, allowing individuals to develop the skills necessary for creating a compassionate future. Positive psychology, on the other hand, helps individuals cultivate hope, optimism and resilience, enabling them to understand their past in a more positive light and build a promising future.

To illustrate the integration of these approaches, imagine a line with zero at the centre (see Fig. 1). At one end of the line is suffering and at the other end is flourishing. Compassion (yin) can only reduce suffering up to a point, while positive psychology (yang) cannot fully address past traumas (Wong, 2012). Both are essential and complementary, creating a balance akin to the yin and yang. If interventions were solely focused on developing happiness and well-being without addressing unresolved trauma, individuals might struggle to move forward. Techniques like 'Three Good Things' (Seligman et al., 2005) are effective but can be enhanced by a compassionate understanding of past experiences. Conversely, focusing solely on reducing suffering may leave individuals at a crossroads, free of immediate distress but lacking direction. Thus, combining compassion and positive psychology provides a holistic approach that not only reduces suffering but also promotes flourishing. For example:

−1: Represents offending and suffering.

0: Represents the absence (desistance) of offending but not necessarily flourishing.

+1: Represents desistance and flourishing.

Focusing solely on well-being might create a 'happy criminal' (Andrews et al., 2011), while only reducing risks without enhancing well-being might not prevent reoffending. This is based on the idea that the absence of suffering does not automatically lead to well-being (Browne et al., 2015; Carruthers & Hood, 2007). Therefore, a balanced approach is needed.

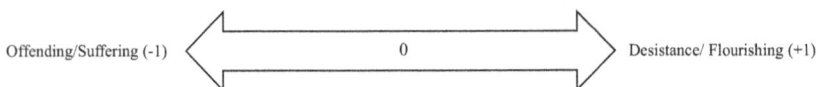

Offending/Suffering (-1)   0   Desistance/ Flourishing (+1)

Fig. 1. The Zero Point.

INTEGRATING COMPASSION AND POSITIVE PSYCHOLOGY

CFT specialises in compassionate motivation to ease distress, addressing the causes (risks) of offending behaviour. Positive psychology aims to improve well-being by fostering positive emotions, strengths and a hopeful outlook on life. By attending to both the causes of offending and future goals, the COMPASS model avoids a hypervigilant focus on relapse prevention and emphasises holistic risk management and life improvement. This approach supports individuals in overcoming substance abuse, personal distress and other low-risk factors, including housing and basic needs.

THE COMPASS MODEL: A HOLISTIC APPROACH

The COMPASS model integrates these elements to support desistance through:

- *Compassion:* Addressing past traumas and shame, creating a foundation for a compassionate future.

- *Positive Psychology:* Promoting hope, optimism and resilience to build a positive outlook on life.

- *Desistance Capital:* Balancing risk reduction and life improvement, addressing both criminogenic needs and personal aspirations.

By combining compassion and positive psychology, the COMPASS model offers a comprehensive framework that supports individuals in transitioning from a state of suffering and offending to one of well-being and flourishing. This integrative approach ensures that both the reduction of risks and the enhancement of well-being are addressed, providing a more effective path to desistance and personal growth.

FEATURES OF THE COMPASS MODEL

The COMPASS model is a holistic model that brings together past experiences, future goals, positive psychology, compassion and desistance capital. It is viewed as a compass with the North representing the future, the East representing compassion, the West positive psychology and the South the past. Each quadrant is divided into sections of a compass but with past compassion/positive psychology (SW, SE) and future compassion and positive psychology

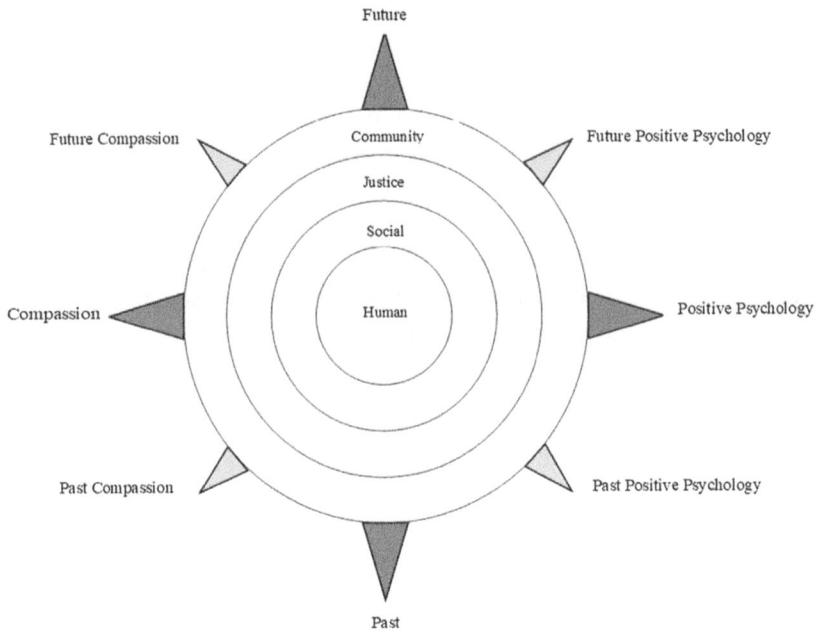

Fig. 2. The COMPASS Model.

(NW, NE). At the centre of the model are four rings that relate to an area of capital (human, social, justice, community) that can help facilitate desistance (see Fig. 2).

THE CARDINAL POINTS OF THE COMPASS MODEL

The past (S) point will be used to focus on what has happened in that person's past, exploring experiences, risks, ACEs and traumas. Past compassion (SE) and positive psychology (SW) will be used to identify when compassion was present or when the individual demonstrated hope, optimism or other strengths that can be built upon going forward. The future compass point (N) is used to identify and create future goals for the individual. Future compassion (NE) and positive psychology (NW) help individuals identify what they would want from each area of desistance capital and develop a compassionate and positive self. This can also be used as a guide for practitioners to choose the most suitable intervention to support their goals and behaviour change. East (E) represents the strengths and skills of compassion and West (W) positive psychology.

THE FOUR INNER RINGS OF DESISTANCE-FOCUSED CAPITAL

The four central rings of desistance-focused capital that sit central to the COMPASS model are associated with the areas of change that can lead to desistance, putting the 'what' into what is needed to make desistance work. In this model, they are human capital, social capital, justice capital and community capital (see Fig. 3). It is important to ensure that for desistance to occur, all types of capital are assessed for and interventions designed to manage any barriers to acquiring desistance capital. For example, working on cognitive skills and having hope for the future is helpful but hindered when there are issues with acquiring housing and employment upon release from prison. Changes in capital can lead to re-offending or desistance from criminal behaviours (Farrall & Maruna, 2004). Even though research explores each area of capital and demonstrates that individually, they can explain the reasons why someone engages in offending, little attention is given to how each combined can influence offender behaviour (Gough & Coghlan, 2022). When united, a person's motivation, skills and social structures that influence their behaviour can be a positive force for supporting change and a lifelong desistance from offending.

Finding our way takes a while, but with the help of the COMPASS, we can keep ourselves on track towards our destination of desistance. This part of the model also acknowledges an integrated system approach where each area of the capital comes together to support and work with the person on their desistance

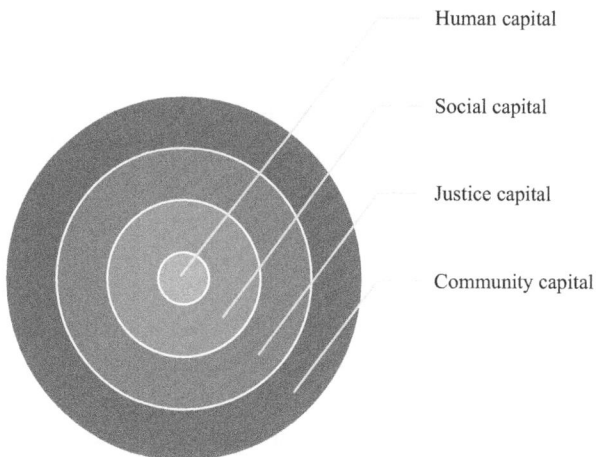

Human capital

Social capital

Justice capital

Community capital

Fig. 3. The Central Rings of Desistance and Criminogenic Focused Capital of the COMPASS Model.

journey. The rings represent a wider radius of trust, support and individual responsibility that spans out in all directions and into infinite opportunities and possibilities. With the person central to this and all other capital around them, they can expand their agentic state through each situational interaction with one of the outer rings. The rings are dynamic in that the person is central but can expand their goals and wants to each other ring. They can draw from each one what they want and need, while each area of capital can provide what the person needs. This helps people who have offended, their social circles, organisations and the wider community come together and work on the same goals and aims to reduce offending behaviour by providing the correct support for each person under the banner of compassion, desistance, strengths and positive psychology. Only when we all come together does desistance happen.

Of course, there will be setbacks in each ring as there is with the process of desistance, but the person can learn from this and, by being gentler to themselves, always return and reorientate in a different direction with what the knowledge gained from each step forward. The aim is to explore each area with the person, consider what enables or hinders them in each capital and seek out effective ways to assist with desistance. To help them broaden their positive repertoire and capital, the rings can be used as both a way to assess and explore what types of capital the offending person has and whether this is persistence or desistance focused and used to support what is needed for the individual. Each area of capital can be viewed as being both a risk for offending and a supportive factor that helps them desist.

HUMAN CAPITAL

At the centre of the rings is human capital because the person wanting to desist is central to all actions of agency and other areas of capital. Human capital includes skills, psychology and personal resources, such as coping mechanisms, resilience, hope and positive aspirations towards a life free of offending. This type of capital is often linked to what is gained through training or higher education and positive problem-solving skills that can be used to help someone develop compassion for self, mental toughness and desist effectively. Human capital includes agency, the internal motivations that the person possesses within them to make change happen and the ability to regulate emotions during the desistance process. It links to primary and secondary desistance and the change in personal identity and behaviour by focusing on identity shifts and who the person wants to be, going forward, and the change in values and pro-social goals they seek to achieve.

Examples of positive human capital include:

- Positive mental health and well-being.

- Addressing learning needs.

- Skill development.

- Pro-social identity, attitudes and behaviours.

- Emotional regulation/self-compassion.

- Cognitive development.

- Distress tolerance.

- Mental Toughness

- Hope and optimism.

- Gratitude.

- Personal agency.

- Problem-solving skills.

SOCIAL CAPITAL

Social capital sits just outside of human capital at the centre and refers to the interpersonal relationships someone has that can either lead to offending behaviour or support them on their desistance journey. It considers the relationships and obligations they have with peers, friends, family or significant others that may have a positive or negative influence on them and lead them either to or away from offending (Best, 2016). For desistance-focused social capital to be effective, a person's commitment and connection to the group must be considered in relation to their bonding and bridging capital (Putnam, 1995). Bonding refers to the strength of the relationship the person has with their social groups and bridging the links they have to other groups and resources that can be used as a way out of offending. Bonding provides strong connections to people who are familiar to us and who can be on hand when we need them for day-to-day needs but fewer opportunities to expand on long-term goals. On the other hand, while the bonds that develop with others are not as strong, bridging allows us to develop dynamic social networks that open us to more experiences that promote goal attainment and increase social status (Putnam, 2000), and like Fredrickson's (2004) Broden and Build theory, more positive experiences open us to opportunities to expand our repertoire and increase well-being. Having access to a range of social networks can increase social support and opportunities, such as finding employment that contributes to desistance-focused social capital. They provide emotional as well as practical support and reduce feelings of isolation.

Examples of positive social capital include:

- Pro-social relationships (family and friends) and other pro-social networks of support.

- Avoidance of pro-criminal groups and peers.

- Access to financial support and other assets that enable the person to integrate back into the community.

JUSTICE CAPITAL

Justice capital is a relatively new addition to the different types of capital that can support people who are desisting from offending and in recovery from addiction. It was introduced to recovery and desistance literature by Best et al. (2021) to highlight the ways in which organisations and the staff that work in them can either help or hinder desistance or re-offending. For example, justice organisations can either provide or prevent access to the resources needed for change. In doing so, these institutions can create the spaces for human, social and community capital to flourish and facilitate desistance or enable offending behaviours to develop further. Examples of positive justice capital include access to training for resilience skills, education, therapeutic care, strengths-based interventions and opportunities for exercise and personal development, in addition to creating spaces that enable social bridging. I would go one further and say they foster the compassionate attitude and understanding that makes people accept and believe in themselves that they can change. An awareness of the risks that can present themselves in a justice setting, such as links to criminal networks, should be considered important for supporting justice capital in the prison system. Each person who works within the criminal justice system has a responsibility to provide the navigational tools and remove all barriers to desistance that lie ahead of the person.

Negative justice capital creates barriers to desistance and is beset by organisations and staff who fail to recognise the needs and challenges of marginalised groups and provide adequate support to provide bridging capital and other factors that aid their recovery, well-being and rehabilitation (Best et al., 2021). Justice organisations are powerful places that have the power to create the spaces for and facilitate change among offenders. Expressing judgement of an offender's crimes creates a negative space between them and the justice worker. When there is no trust, the relationship between staff and offenders breaks down, leading to more problems and fewer resources for desistance to happen (Best et al., 2021).

Examples of positive justice capital include:

- Trauma-informed staff and approaches to offending behaviour.

- Compassion is central to all approaches and interactions with people desisting.

- Positive values and beliefs from staff that change is possible.

- Become models of hope and optimism.

- Working with other organisations to build capital and resources that support the person's desistance.

- A compassionate understanding of the challenges faced by people who have offended and the people who work with them, such as stigma and other barriers to other forms of desistance capital.

- Accountability of the criminal justice organisations and those who work in them to do their job compassionately and with the firm belief that desistance and positive change are positive.

- Communication that is based on understanding (use of interpreter where needed).

COMMUNITY CAPITAL

Community capital is the outer ring because it focuses on the wider community resources that are available and can be used to support desistance. It links with tertiary desistance and one's sense of belonging to a pro-social community (McNeill, 2016). Social bridging and bonding can also influence community capital through the moral connections that are made by accessing these resources.

Community capital contains, within it, cultural capital, as the communities from which people come or turn are very much a part of the fabric of that community. They are the people who can make some of the person's needs become reality or give them a place to feel part of something and gain meaning from it. Having a stable home is crucial for desistance and can be achieved with positive community capital. An example of this is the local authority that helps make sure someone has a decent home to live in upon release from prison, such as providing people on probation with financial support to improve their living conditions (Wilfong et al., 2021). Food banks and employment agencies are other community resources that are much needed to support people desisting from offending. Community engagement in activities and events that promote and help sustain desistance play a significant role in preventing recidivism. At the policy level, government initiatives which create supportive community environments and organisations that promote desistance from offending are necessary. For example, providing funding for organisations and groups that provide crucial support to gain access to help with things like housing, addiction and finding work without feeling stigmatised for having a criminal record. It is the places the person can join, such as a gym, to improve their physical health and well-being. The place that creates a sense of connection, belonging and meaning in the community (Thompson & Spacey, 2023) and provides social support which helps reduce criminal thinking and the development of a pro-social identity (Duwe & Johnson, 2023). Educational organisations such as universities that give people a chance to change through education and the success of gaining a degree, master's or PhD, and then meaningful employment are also helpful. All the external factors, people and places are part of the fabric of real and effective change that empowers the person central to the change.

Examples of positive community capital include access to:

- Suitable and supportive housing to help with reintegration into the community.

- Educational and employment opportunities and recourses to develop skills and abilities.

- Places of worship, spiritual, religious and cultural environments that support meaning and social connection.

- Health and well-being such as gyms and other sports and recreational activities that enable pro-social connections in the community and the improvement of physical and mental well-being.

IMPLICATIONS FOR RESEARCH, POLICY AND PRACTICE

Barnao and Ward (2015) spoke of the challenges of trying to navigate the uncharted seas of forensic mental health without a compass. For justice practitioners, the COMPASS model serves as a framework with a set of guiding principles and practices that can be applied to intervention design for justice-involved people to aid in the understanding of why they have offended and how they can be assisted on their desistance journey. Because of the nature of the work they do, practitioners can also use the ideas presented in the model to support themselves. For people desisting, the model provides knowledge of effective strategies that they can use to map out a path towards their desistance goals. Researchers can use the model to develop new knowledge and understanding of what works to help people desist from offending. At the policy level, it can act as a framework for considering the varying systems people find themselves in how they affect crime rates, and what we can do to reduce them.

The COMPASS model can be tailored to targeted, universal and specialist interventions to aid with desistance (Kemshall, 2021). It can be used with specific sub-groups of offenders, such as young, female, persistent and sexual offenders. It can also be applied to the universal needs of service users and support compassionate and positive thinking skills, accommodation and employment needs. It is applicable to high-, medium- and low-risk offenders and can be adjusted to fit their individual needs. Furthermore, interventions can be adapted for people with complex mental health and substance use needs (Best et al., 2021). The COMPASS model could be used to decide what the best course of action is for someone who has offended. For example, assessing whether prison or a community-based punishment is more suitable for the offence. It can guide decision-makers on the direct of the person's life and towards interventions that aim to reduce offending and support desistance.

CONCLUSION

The COMPASS model integrates essential elements from CFT and positive psychology, blending them with the concept of desistance capital. By incorporating insights from the Risk-Need-Responsivity (RNR) model and the Good Lives Model (GLM), the COMPASS model addresses the risks and needs associated with offending while emphasising positive goals and aspirations for those on the path to desistance. The model aims to explore and mitigate risk factors through a compassionate perspective, promoting pro-social living and addressing past traumas. It evaluates both historical causes of offending and current needs for desistance, providing a comprehensive framework for individuals seeking to leave behind criminal behaviours and for practitioners supporting them. By examining the past, present and future, the COMPASS model offers a holistic view that helps individuals and practitioners understand the broader context of desistance and motivation. This approach not only guides individuals in their journey towards a crime-free future but also assists professionals in facilitating and supporting this transformation. In the final chapter, I will present two case studies that illustrate the application of the COMPASS model with individuals who have lived experience of the criminal justice system. These case studies will provide evidence of the model's effectiveness and demonstrate its practical impact.

REFERENCES

Andrews, D. A., Bonta, J., & Wormith, J. S. (2011). The risk-need-responsivity (RNR) model: Does adding the good lives model contribute to effective crime prevention? *Criminal Justice and Behavior, 38*(7), 735–755.

Barnao, M., & Ward, T. (2015). Sailing uncharted seas without a compass: A review of interventions in forensic mental health. *Aggression and Violent Behavior, 22,* 77–86.

Best, D. (2016). Social identity, social networks and social capital in desistance and recovery. In A. Robinson & P. Hamilton (Eds.), *Moving on from crime and substance use* (pp. 175–194). Policy Press.

Best, D., Hamilton, S., Hall, L., & Bartels, L. (2021). Justice capital: A model for reconciling structural and agentic determinants of desistance. *Probation Journal, 68*(2), 206–223.

Browne, C., Notkin, S., Schneider-Muñoz, A., & Zimmerman, F. (2015). Youth thrive: A framework to help adolescents overcome trauma and thrive. *Journal of Child and Youth Care Work, 25,* 33–52.

Carruthers, C. P., & Hood, C. D. (2007). Building a life of meaning through therapeutic recreation: The leisure and well-being model, part I. *Therapeutic Recreation Journal, 41*(4), 276.

Duwe, G., & Johnson, B. R. (2023). New insights for "what works"? Religiosity and the risk-needs-responsivity model. *Crime & Delinquency.* https://doi.org/10.1177/00111287231160736

Farrall, S., & Maruna, S. (2004). Desistance-focused criminal justice policy research: Introduction to a special issue on desistance from crime and public policy. *The Howard Journal of Criminal Justice, 43*(4), 358–367.

Fredrickson, B. L. (2004). The broaden–and–build theory of positive emotions. *Philosophical Transactions of the Royal Society of London. Series B: Biological Sciences, 359*(1449), 1367–1377.

Gough, D., & Coghlan, M. (2022). *Understanding reoffending: Push factors and preventative responses.* University of Portsmouth. https://assets.gov.ie/239978/75a21996-0062-405b-8a45-366ac01e8306.pdf

Kemshall, H. (2021). *Risk and desistance: A blended approach to risk management* (Vol. 7). HM Inspectorate of Probation Academic Insights.

McNeill, F. (2016). Desistance and criminal justice in Scotland. In H. Croall, G. Mooney, & R. Munro (Eds.), *Crime, justice, and society in Scotland* (pp. 200–216). Routledge.

Moore, C., & Gino, F. (2013). Ethically adrift: How others pull our moral compass from true North, and how we can fix it. *Research in Organizational Behavior, 33*, 53–77.

Putnam, R. D. (1995). Bowling alone: America's declining social capital. *Journal of Democracy, 6*(1), 65–78. https://doi.org/10.1353/jod.1995.0002

Putnam, R. (2000). *Bowling alone: The collapse and revival of American community.* Simon & Schuster.

Seligman, M. E. P., Steen, T. A., Park, N., & Peterson, C. (2005). Positive psychology progress: Empirical validation of interventions. *American Psychologist, 60*, 410–421.

Thompson, N., & Spacey, M. (2023). "I would want to see young people working in here, that's what I want to see..." How peer support opportunities in youth offending services can support a Child First, trauma-informed, and reparative model of practice for youth justice. *Safer Communities, 22*(3), 200–216.

Van Gelder, J. L., Cornet, L. J., Zwalua, N. P., Mertens, E. C., & van der Schalk, J. (2022). Interaction with the future self in virtual reality reduces self-defeating behavior in a sample of convicted offenders. *Scientific Reports*, 12(1), 2254.

Wilfong, J., Golder, S., Logan, T. K., & Higgins, G. (2021). Examining the influence of financial assistance and employment services on the criminal justice outcomes of women on probation. *Affilia*, 36(2), 240–253.

Wong, P. T. P. (2012). Toward a dual-systems model of what makes life worth living. In P. T. P. Wong (Ed.), *The human quest for meaning: Theories, research, and applications* (2nd ed., pp. 3–22). Routledge.

8

ASSESSING THE COMPASS MODEL

ABSTRACT

This chapter examines the strengths of the Compassionate Positive Applied Strengths-based Solutions (COMPASS) model in the context of desistance capital, using historical case studies to illustrate how the model's principles have facilitated successful desistance and recovery journeys. By integrating research on compassion and positive psychology within offender populations, this chapter underscores the effectiveness of the COMPASS model. Through detailed examples, it aims to validate the model's approach, offering insights and recommendations for future practices in the justice system.

Keywords: COMPASS; capital; staff well-being; assessment; evidence; compassionate approach

EVIDENCING THE LINKS BETWEEN DESISTANCE CAPITAL AND INTERVENTIONAL APPROACHES OF THE COGNITIVE BEHAVIOURAL THERAPY (COMPASS) MODEL

The COMPASS model, though novel in its application, draws on established theories and practices in compassion and positive psychology that have demonstrated effectiveness in reducing offending and enhancing well-being. This section explores how the COMPASS model integrates with desistance capital and supports the process of desistance through evidence and practical examples.

HUMAN/PSYCHOLOGICAL CAPITAL: UNDERSTANDING HUMAN CAPITAL AND NARRATIVE IDENTITY

Human capital involves the cognitive, emotional and psychological resources an individual brings to the desistance process. A critical element of this is narrative identity, which encompasses how individuals perceive their past, present and future selves. If an individual struggles to envision a non-offending identity due to restrictive social structures or self-limiting beliefs, they may experience learned helplessness and persist in their deviant identity (Liu & Bachman, 2021). Addressing these barriers through a compassionate under-standing of past traumas, such as abuse, can be pivotal in facilitating cognitive and identity transformation.

Positive Psychological Interventions (PPI) have been effective in shifting criminal thinking towards a more optimistic and pro-social mindset. PPIs help individuals focus on their strengths, foster gratitude and build social and community capital, all of which contribute to desistance (Ang, 2016). These interventions improve life satisfaction, reduce aggression and address crimi-nogenic risk factors (Deng et al., 2019; Woldgabreal et al., 2016). When combined with Cognitive Behavioural Therapy (CBT), PPIs enhance well-being and alleviate symptoms of mental health issues like depression and anxiety (Mak & Chan, 2018). Compassion directed towards oneself also plays a significant role. It can mitigate feelings of shame and reduce aggression by promoting self-control and empathy (Dávila Gómez et al., 2020; Hofmann & Jeffries, 2022). Self-compassion helps individuals manage their shame and guilt, facilitating self-acceptance and release from internal barriers that may hinder desistance (Taylor, 2021). Compassion-Focused Therapy (CFT) has proven effective in reducing psychopathic traits and disruptive behaviours, supporting those with sexual offences in understanding their actions and making sense of their backgrounds (Ribeiro da Silva et al., 2019; Rousseau et al., 2019).

SOCIAL CAPITAL: BUILDING PRO-SOCIAL SOCIAL CAPITAL

Effective desistance requires the development and reinforcement of pro-social bonds and the identification of supportive networks. For individuals tran-sitioning out of offending, strengthening connections with desistance-focused groups and bridging opportunities is crucial (Sapouna et al., 2015). For those previously involved in criminal networks or coming from criminogenic environments, moving away from these ties can be challenging due to entrenched social bonds. Self-compassion is linked to lower criminal impulsivity and more positive social connections, which are critical for desistance (Morley et al., 2016). Positive social relationships enhance meaning, purpose and a sense of belonging, further supporting desistance (Vanhooren et al., 2016). High levels of meaning are associated with increased care and compassion for others, reduced distress and improved self-worth.

JUSTICE CAPITAL: CREATING TRUST AND COMPASSION IN JUSTICE SETTINGS

Justice practitioners can foster trust and protect individuals from anti-social influences by adopting a compassionate and positive approach. This approach should extend to all personnel involved in the justice system, including prison staff, probation officers, healthcare workers and therapists. Compassion and positive psychology can enhance case management and relationships within the justice system, promoting growth and hope (Cross et al., 2012; Lai et al., 2021). For example, research shows that compassionate interactions between prison officers and inmates can reduce emotional responses and foster a shared sense of humanity (DeCelles & Anteby, 2020; Hammarström et al., 2019). Similarly, compassion in forensic nursing helps staff manage emotional vulnerability and respond effectively to patients' needs (Hammarström et al., 2020). Such compassionate approaches are integral to developing effective therapeutic relationships and supporting desistance.

PRACTITIONER SKILLS AND STAFF WELL-BEING: ENHANCING PRACTITIONER SKILLS AND SUPPORTING WELL-BEING

Practitioners' attitudes and skills are crucial for implementing the COMPASS model. Compassion training equips staff to view individuals in the justice system with empathy and respect, avoiding judgement based on their offences. This approach fosters a therapeutic relationship grounded in common humanity and support for personal change. Given the emotional demands of working in justice settings, it is essential to address staff well-being. Compassion practices can mitigate burnout and secondary trauma, promoting resilience and morale among staff. Training in compassion and positive psychology helps students and practitioners manage stress and maintain a compassionate stance towards themselves and their clients (Beaumont et al., 2016; Durkin et al., 2016; Spaan et al., 2024).

COMMUNITY CAPITAL: FOSTERING COMMUNITY CONNECTIONS

Practitioners can help individuals build community connections that support their desistance journey. Engaging with community-based interventions and spiritual gatherings can enhance community capital and improve well-being (Geary et al., 2005; Mapham & Hefferon, 2012). Positive psychology programmes, such as those which encourage community involvement and spiritual participation, facilitate pro-social relationships and increase optimism, aiding in the desistance process (Duan et al., 2024).

The COMPASS model's integration of compassion and positive psychology with desistance capital provides a robust framework for supporting individuals in their journey away from offending. By addressing human, social, justice and community capital through compassionate and positive practices, the model offers a comprehensive approach to facilitating desistance and improving well-being.

A COMPASS APPROACH TO WORKING WITH SOMEONE DESISTING FROM OFFENDING

The COMPASS approach to desistance is designed to integrate compassion and positive psychology into the process of helping individuals transition away from offending. This approach acknowledges the complexity of each person's journey and aims to address their needs through a comprehensive and compassionate framework. Here's a detailed guide on how to apply the COMPASS model, focusing on the past, present and future aspects of the individual's life.

KEY PRINCIPLES OF THE COMPASS APPROACH

- *Compassionate Understanding*: Recognise that individuals are more than their offences. They are human beings with complex histories, including traumatic experiences, disabilities and socio-economic challenges. A compassionate approach helps build a therapeutic relationship and acknowledges our common humanity.

- *Holistic View of Desistance*: Consider the person's entire life context, including past traumas, current needs and future aspirations. This helps in creating a supportive environment where individuals feel understood and motivated to change.

- *Positive Strengths-Focused*: Acknowledge and work with the persons strengths with hope, optimism and belief in the future.

ASSESSMENT AND FORMULATION PROCESS

The assessment process involves three stages and is based on the COMPASS model where South is past experiences and risks, North is future goals and needs and East and West are the compassion based and positive psychology interventions that are used to assist in the desistance journey. The central rings represent the different types of capital someone has or wants to work on that can support them going forward. It can be used with people who have offended and with staff to identify potential issues that are causing stress-related burnout and fatigue.

Past

- *Gathering Background Information*: Collect detailed information about the person's past experiences, including traumatic events, ACEs socio-economic factors and personal strengths. Understand the risk factors and capital that have shaped their behaviour. Identify collaborative and factors that contributed to offending, such as addiction, unstable family environments or exposure to violence.

- *Exploring Strengths*: Identify the strengths and resilience the person has demonstrated despite past adversities. Recognise their ability to overcome obstacles as a foundation for their desistance journey.

- *Compassionate reflection*: Use compassionate language and non-judgemental approaches to help the person revisit their past experiences. Create a safe space for them to explore their life story without blame or shame. Focus on feelings of guilt rather than shame. This shift can foster a sense of responsibility and motivation for change. Help the person reframe their life story through a compassionate lens. Use timelines, drawings or other creative methods to reflect on past experiences and understand them in a non-judgemental way.

Present

- *Understanding current capital*: Assess the person's current psychological, social and justice capital. This includes their mental health status, social support network and any existing barriers to desistance.

- *Exploring goals and motivation*: Discuss their present goals and aspirations. Identify what they want to change in their life and the motivations driving these desires. Align their current resources and strengths with their goals.

- *Strengths and Challenges*: Identify strengths that can aid in desistance and challenges that may need to be addressed, such as ongoing addiction issues or lack of stable housing.

Future

- *Creating a Future Plan*: Develop a comprehensive plan for the future, including specific, achievable goals. Create a visual map of the steps needed to achieve future goals. Include specific dates and potential obstacles and revise the map as necessary to adapt to changing circumstances. Use tools like pathway mapping to outline steps towards these goals and anticipate potential obstacles (Feldman & Dreher, 2012; Snyder, 1994). Identify interventions and support mechanisms needed to achieve these goals. This could include therapy, vocational training or substance abuse treatment.

- *Best Possible Self Exercise*: Engage in exercises that help visualise an optimistic future. Writing or drawing about their best possible self can increase positive emotions and motivation (Carrillo et al., 2019). This can be done in collaboration with Creating a Future Plan.

- *Optimising Goals and Pathways*: Set realistic timelines and strategies for achieving goals. Define clear, achievable goals for the future. This includes personal aspirations, career objectives and social reintegration plans. Incorporate strategies to overcome anticipated obstacles and revise the plan as needed. Develop a step-by-step plan to reach these goals, including short-term and long-term actions. For example, enrolling in educational programmes, seeking employment, finding housing or joining community groups.

- *Future Capital*: Explore future capital and encourage the person to consider what they need going forward that will assist them with their desistance.

- *Obstacles and Solutions*: Anticipate potential obstacles and strategies, solutions to overcome them. This helps maintain motivation and stay on track.

POINTS TO CONSIDER WHEN USING ASSESSMENT AND FORMULATION

A COMPASS approach to assessment and formulation involves understanding the person's life experiences and mapping out a positive future. It should focus on:

- *Collaborative Approach*: Engage the person in a co-formulation process. Work together to understand their past, identify their strengths and barriers and plan for a different future. It should be a step-by-step process, allowing for gradual exploration of past experiences, the present and future goals. This ensures that the plan reflects the individual's personal experiences, goals and needs. Regular meetings can be held to review progress, adjust goals and adapt the plan as necessary. This helps manage emotional responses and maintain engagement.

- *Positive Compassionate Language*: Avoid diagnostic or judgemental language. The goal is not to diagnose but to use compassionate and understanding language to explain past behaviours, present situations and support future changes. Avoid terms that might induce shame or blame, focusing instead on how past experiences have shaped their behaviour. Hopeful and honest terminology can install belief in the person that change is possible.

- *Avoidance and Approach Goals*: Balance avoidance of risk factors with the development of pro-social behaviours. Help the person recognise what needs to be avoided and what new opportunities can be pursued.

- *Creative Expression*: Use narrative or visual methods to help the person articulate their life story and future aspirations. This can include timelines, drawings or written narratives.

- *Strength-Based Exploration*: Identify and leverage the person's strengths and resilience. Explore how they have used these strengths in the past and how they can be applied to future goals.

- *The COMPASS MAP is not static*: It can be revised and updated as circumstances change. This flexibility allows the individual to continually adapt their plan to reflect new insights and challenges.

By combining compassion and positive psychology with a structured approach to assessing and planning, the COMPASS model offers a comprehensive framework for supporting individuals in their journey away from offending. This approach helps individuals understand their past, leverage their strengths, make sense of different levels of capital that can either hinder or help in the present and create a hopeful and achievable path to a desistance-focused future.

The main objectives of the COMPASS interventions are:

- *Provide Trauma-Informed Support*: To ensure that interventions are sensitive to the individual's past traumas and experiences. This involves understanding how trauma has shaped their behaviour and providing support that acknowledges and addresses these underlying issues.

- *Personalised Approach*: To tailor interventions based on the individual's unique life story, current circumstances and future aspirations. This requires a thorough assessment of their past experiences, present needs, and future goals to create a comprehensive and individualised plan.

- *Compassion-Based Practice*: To use CFT and positive psychology to address emotional and psychological issues. CFT helps manage anger and emotional regulation by addressing deep-seated issues sensitively, while positive psychology fosters strengths and resilience.

- *Goal Setting and Mapping*: To work collaboratively with individuals to set realistic and achievable desistance goals. This involves creating a COMPASS MAP that outlines steps towards these goals, identifies potential obstacles and integrates strategies for overcoming them.

- *Enhance Well-being*: To promote overall well-being through interventions that increase hope, optimism and life satisfaction. This includes using positive psychology techniques to envision and work towards a pro-social future that improves the quality of life.

- *Build Resilience*: To strengthen the individual's resilience by helping them understand and leverage their strengths. This involves exploring how they have overcome past challenges and applying these insights to their desistance journey.

- *Foster Agency and Control*: To empower individuals by helping them recognise their capacity to influence their future. This includes encouraging a sense of agency and control over their life choices and desistance path.

- *Create Pro-Social Capital and Support Networks*: To identify and strengthen supportive relationships and community connections. This involves connecting individuals with pro-social networks and resources that can aid in their desistance and integration into society.

By focusing on these objectives, COMPASS interventions aim to provide a holistic, compassionate and practical framework for supporting individuals in their journey away from offending and towards a fulfilling and pro-social life.

THE COMPASS MY ALTERNATIVE PATH (MAP)

The COMPASS MAP is a collaborative planning tool designed to assist individuals in their desistance journey by mapping out their past, present and future. It can be utilised at various stages, whether during incarceration or in the community, to chart a course away from offending behaviour and towards a positive and sustainable future. The MAP allows the individual and practitioner to work together to identify past influences, current challenges and future goals, ultimately helping to create a comprehensive plan for change. It can be used *During Incarceration* where an individual might use the MAP to set educational and personal development goals while in prison, such as working on their emotional regulation or participating in vocational training programmes. At *Post-Release* and *In the Community*, the MAP can then be used to plan for reintegration into the community, including finding housing, securing employment and building supportive relationships. By working together with a practitioner, individuals can create a personalised and actionable plan that addresses their unique needs and aspirations.

Below (Table 3) is an example of how the COMPASS MAP might be completed for someone who has just been released from prison.

Table 3. An Example of a Completed COMPASS MAP.

Capital	Past – what are the risks/experiences that have led to offending. Risks- High/Med/ Low ACEs	Present – where are they now/what do they need in the moment. What is motivating them to change. Risks – High/Med/Low ACES	Future – what are the goals that can help facilitate desistance/what do they want/need
Human	Previous trauma Addiction to cope	Determined to stop relying on drugs to manage feelings	To become resilient and drug free Build on strengths
Social	Anti-social friends – drug taking	Has supportive family willing to help	To avoid past friends and strengthen bonds with pro-social friends and family
Community	Lack of opportunity No fixed abode	Needs a place to stay – housing	To have a home Go to gym Volunteer at local charity – help others
Justice	Lack of support from local authority to help with drug addiction	Drugs counsellor/worker	
COMPASS plan	• Compassion-based therapy and intervention understand underlying causes of drug use. • Develop COMPASS life plan – ideal self, gratitude, self-compassion. • Speak to family about living accommodation and support. • Find suitable housing. • Look et employment opportunities.		

STORIES OF CHANGE AND DESISTANCE UNDERPINNED BY COMPASS PRINCIPLES

The following stories are based on real-life experiences of people who have desisted from crime guided by the principles of the COMPASS model. The names have been changed to protect their anonymity.

SAM'S JOURNEY TO DESISTANCE

Background

Sam (not her real name), a 35-year-old female, grew up in a challenging environment marked by substance abuse, family violence and poverty. Her early years were shaped by exposure to physical and emotional abuse, which led her into a cycle of drug addiction and criminal behaviour.

Past

Sam's childhood was turbulent. Her father was an abusive alcoholic, and her mother struggled with severe mental health issues, leaving Sam to fend for herself. By the age of 15, Sam was deeply involved in drug use, which provided a temporary escape from her traumatic home life. She quickly became entangled in criminal activities, including theft and drug dealing, to support her addiction. The repeated cycles of arrest and incarceration only deepened her sense of hopelessness and despair.

Present

After several years of incarceration and failed rehabilitation attempts, Sam encountered a pivotal moment during a prison therapy programme. Here, she was introduced to CFT and positive psychology principles. Initially sceptical, Sam gradually embraced these approaches with the help of a dedicated counsellor who demonstrated genuine compassion and belief in her potential for change. Through CFT, Sam began addressing her deep-seated trauma and internalised shame. She learned to develop self-compassion, recognising the impact of his past experiences without letting them define her future. Positive psychology interventions helped Sam cultivate hope and optimism, focusing on her strengths and setting achievable goals. She engaged in a distance learning educational programme, completed a degree in social work and participated in group therapy sessions that emphasised building a supportive network.

Future

Sam's transformation has been profound. Having completed her sentence, she now works as a social worker helping others from similar backgrounds, a profession she feels allows her to give back to the community. Sam actively participates in a community support group for individuals recovering from addiction and gives talks at local schools about her experiences, aiming to prevent youth from falling into similar traps. She maintains a strong focus on her well-being through regular mindfulness practices and therapy sessions, continually reinforcing her self-compassion and positive outlook. Sam also volunteers with a local organisation that supports victims of abuse, using his experiences to offer guidance and hope to others in similar situations.

Sam's journey from a life of addiction and crime to one of stability and purpose illustrates the transformative power of compassion and positive psychology. Her story underscores the importance of addressing trauma with compassion and providing individuals with the tools to envision and achieve a positive future. Through her commitment to personal growth and community support, Sam exemplifies the potential for profound change and desistance from a life of offending.

MARK'S JOURNEY TO DESISTANCE

Mark was a 30-year-old male, who experienced great loss from an early age and struggled to find meaning and purpose in his life. Through access to various forms of capital, compassion, hope and belief, he was able to turn his life around and go from being imprisoned for drug dealing offences to a PhD in psychology and published author.

Past

Mark grew up in a loving family but never knew his father. This absence hurt him deeply and fuelled a lingering anger. School was a traumatic experience for him. In primary school, teachers dismissed his potential, and secondary school offered no reprieve. These formative years were marred by the death of many friends, which profoundly impacted his worldview, confidence and sense of self. Life seemed pointless. Mark struggled with his identity and purpose, finding temporary solace in raves, ecstasy and the fleeting moments spent with the few friends he had left. The combination of loss and drug use forged a strong bond with those around him, and taking drugs became a regular part of his life. This gradual normalisation of drug use led him to dealing, which provided him with a sense of identity and purpose. With limited education and job prospects, Mark turned to selling party drugs as a means of making money and enjoying life. This quickly escalated to dealing harder drugs until, at 19, he was caught and sentenced to five and a half years in prison, eventually being released on probation after serving half his sentence.

Present

Upon his release, Mark struggled to reintegrate into society and find meaningful work. His search for identity continued, leading to further trouble and two more charges related to violent behaviour, though he was fortunate to receive probation. While in prison, Mark had attended some psychology classes that sparked his interest, but the idea of pursuing higher education felt daunting due to his limited academic background. However, after a decade of drifting from job to job with little hope for the future, a chance encounter with a careers advisor at a local library revealed an opportunity. Mark learned about a university course that could provide the qualifications he needed to study psychology at a degree level.

Future

Mark applied to the course and excelled, which significantly boosted his self-belief and motivated him to pursue further education. Over the next 10 years, he not only graduated with a first-class degree in counselling psychology but also completed a master's and eventually a PhD in psychology. His research focused on compassion and positive psychology in healthcare staff, allowing him to apply both theory and practice to his life experiences. This helped him make sense of his past and understand what had kept him motivated to succeed. The support from friends, university staff and others within his social and community networks played a crucial role in changing his outlook on life and fostering self-belief. Mark is proud to have finally developed a strong sense of self and a new, pro-social identity. Most importantly, he has completely desisted from offending.

Mark's story aligns with the COMPASS model, in which he expanded his overall pro-social capital and well-being through education and community connections. He also developed the skills of compassion, resilience, optimism and hope, which helped him regulate his emotions and find meaning in his life.

CONCLUSION

This chapter has provided compelling evidence for the COMPASS model, supported by extensive literature on compassion and positive psychology, particularly in relation to capital and its role in promoting desistance among offenders. The case studies further reinforce the effectiveness of the COMPASS approach, offering concrete examples of its impact. The COMPASS model not only builds on evidence-based practices in Forensic and Criminal Psychology, capital and desistance but also draws deeply from criminology and, crucially, the author's own lived experience within the criminal justice system. This model doesn't just advocate for what works, it explains how it works and underscores the importance of integrating compassion theory and positive psychology to explore past experiences, navigate present challenges and shape future pathways for those seeking to desist from crime. Incorporating the concept of capital within this framework helps individuals who have offended, as well as those who support them, to identify their strengths and the specific resources they need to move forward. It also highlights potential obstacles, supporting primary, secondary and tertiary desistance. In doing so, the COMPASS model focuses as much on the needs of the individual as it does on the risks they may pose to the community. This book speaks directly to those who matter most, the individuals who have offended. The author's lived experience of the justice system and a profound belief in the possibility of change aim to inspire and empower these individuals. It sends a clear message: if one person can successfully navigate the journey of desistance, then anyone can. They too can become leaders in their own journey, paving the way for others to follow, or at the very least, sharing their stories to foster hope that change is within reach for everyone.

As we conclude, I want to leave you with a sense of optimism for the future, one that can be shared with every person who has offended and wants to desist. We all may lose our way at times, but with the right tools, a positive strengths-based approach, kinder understanding of ourselves and others and, of course, a COMPASS, we can find our way again. I am living proof of this and firmly believe that anyone, given the right support, can ultimately reach a life free of offending.

REFERENCES

Ang, X. (2016). *Positive psychology intervention for girls with conduct problems: A single-case time-series design.* The University of Alabama.

Beaumont, E., Durkin, M., Hollins Martin, C. J., & Carson, J. (2016). Measuring relationships between self-compassion, compassion fatigue, burnout and well-being in student counsellors and student cognitive behavioural psychotherapists: A quantitative survey. *Counselling and Psychotherapy Research*, *16*(1), 15–23.

Carrillo, A., Rubio-Aparicio, M., Molinari, G., Enrique, A., Sanchez-Meca, J., & Banos, R. M. (2019). Effects of the best possible self-intervention: A systematic review and meta-analysis. *PLoS One*, *14*(9), e0222386.

Cross, L. E., Morrison, W., Peterson, P., & Domene, J. F. (2012). Investigating positive psychology approaches in case management and residential programming with incarcerated youth. *Canadian Journal of Counselling and Psychotherapy*, *46*(2).

Dávila Gómez, M., Dávila Pino, J., & Dávila Pino, R. (2020). Self-compassion and predictors of criminal conduct in adolescent offenders. *Journal of Aggression, Maltreatment & Trauma*, *29*(8), 1020–1033.

DeCelles, K. A., & Anteby, M. (2020). Compassion in the clink: When and how human services workers overcome barriers to care. *Organization Science*, *31*(6), 1408–1431.

Deng, Y., Xiang, R., Zhu, Y., Li, Y., Yu, S., & Liu, X. (2019). Counting blessings and sharing gratitude in a Chinese prisoner sample: Effects of gratitude-based interventions on subjective well-being and aggression. *The Journal of Positive Psychology*, *14*(3), 303–311.

Duan, W., Wang, Z., Yang, C., & Ke, S. (2024). Are risk-need-responsivity principles golden? A meta-analysis of randomized controlled trials of community correction programs. *Journal of Experimental Criminology*, *20*(2), 593–616.

Durkin, M., Beaumont, E., Martin, C. J. H., & Carson, J. (2016). A pilot study exploring the relationship between self-compassion, self-judgement, self-kindness, compassion, professional quality of life and wellbeing among UK community nurses. *Nurse Education Today*, *46*, 109–114.

Feldman, D. B., & Dreher, D. E. (2012). Can hope be changed in 90 minutes? Testing the efficacy of a single-session goal-pursuit intervention for college students. *Journal of Happiness Studies*, *13*, 745–759.

Geary, B., Ciarrocchi, J. W., & Scheers, N. J. (2005). Spirituality and religious variables as predictors of well-being in sex offenders. In *Research in the social scientific study of religion* (Vol. 15). Brill. https://doi.org/10.1163/9789047406563_013

Hammarström, L., Devik, S. A., Hellzén, O., & Häggström, M. (2020). The path of compassion in forensic psychiatry. *Archives of Psychiatric Nursing, 34*(6), 435–441.

Hammarström, L., Häggström, M., Devik, S. A., & Hellzen, O. (2019). Controlling emotions: Nurses' lived experiences caring for patients in forensic psychiatry. *International Journal of Qualitative Studies on Health and Well-Being, 14*(1), 1682911.

Hofmann, S. A., & Jeffries, Z. J. (2022). Self-compassion as a potential mediator of shame and aggression in youth offenders. *International Journal of Criminal Justice Sciences, 17*(2), 1–14.

Lai, A. Y. K., Sit, S. M. M., Thomas, C., Cheung, G. O. C., Wan, A., Chan, S. S. C., & Lam, T. H. (2021). A randomized controlled trial of a positive family holistic health intervention for probationers in Hong Kong: A mixed-methods study. *Frontiers in Psychology, 12*, 739418.

Liu, L., & Bachman, R. (2021). Self-identity and persistent offending: A quantitative test of identity theory of desistance. *Journal of Offender Rehabilitation, 60*(5), 341–357.

Mak, V. W., & Chan, C. K. (2018). Effects of cognitive-behavioural therapy (CBT) and positive psychological intervention (PPI) on female offenders with psychological distress in Hong Kong. *Criminal Behaviour and Mental Health, 28*(2), 158–173.

Mapham, A., & Hefferon, K. (2012). "I used to be an offender, now I'm a defender": Positive psychology approaches in the facilitation of posttraumatic growth in offenders. *Journal of Offender Rehabilitation, 51*(6), 389–413.

Morley, R. M., Terranova, V. A., Cunningham, S. N., & Kraft, G. (2016). Self-compassion and predictors of criminality. *Journal of Aggression, Maltreatment & Trauma, 25*(5), 503–517.

Ribeiro da Silva, D., Rijo, D., Castilho, P., & Gilbert, P. (2019). The efficacy of a compassion-focused therapy-based intervention in reducing psychopathic traits and disruptive behaviour: A clinical case study with a juvenile detainee. *Clinical Case Studies, 18*(5), 323–343.

Rousseau, D., Long, N., Jackson, E., & Jurgensen, J. (2019). Empowering through embodied awareness: Evaluation of a peer-facilitated trauma-informed mindfulness curriculum in a woman's prison. *The Prison Journal, 99*(Suppl. 4), 14S–37S.

Sapouna, M., Bisset, C., Conlong, A. M., & Matthews, B. (2015). *What works to reduce reoffending: A summary of the evidence.* Scottish Government Social Research.

Snyder, C. R. (1994). *The psychology of hope: You can get there from here.* Free Press.

Spaan, P., van den Boogert, F., Bouman, Y. H., Hoogendijk, W. J., & Roza, S. J. (2024). How are you coping? Stress, coping, burnout, and aggression in forensic mental healthcare workers. *Frontiers in Psychology, 14,* 1301878.

Taylor, J. (2021). Compassion in custody: Developing a trauma sensitive intervention for men with developmental disabilities who have convictions for sexual offending. *Advances in Mental Health and Intellectual Disabilities, 15*(5), 185–200.

Vanhooren, S., Leijssen, M., & Dezutter, J. (2016). Profiles of meaning and search for meaning among prisoners. *The Journal of Positive Psychology, 11*(6), 622–633.

Woldgabreal, Y., Day, A., & Ward, T. (2016). Linking positive psychology to offender supervision outcomes: The mediating role of psychological flexibility, general self-efficacy, optimism, and hope. *Criminal Justice and Behaviour, 43*(6), 697–721.

ABOUT THE AUTHOR

Mark A. Durkin is a Lecturer in Psychology at Leeds Trinity University. His main research interests include compassion and positive psychology and how both can be applied to support people's mental health and well-being and help them manage work-related stress and past traumas, with a specific focus on those with justice experience. He has lived experience of the UK justice system and combines this with his knowledge of Compassionate Mind Training, Positive Psychology, Desistance and Capital Theory to create the Compassionate Positive Applied Strengths-based Solutions (COMPASS) model. In addition to this, he volunteers with others in the world of sport, and youth support, incorporating the ideas of the COMPASS model to help them find their way and flourish.